ABOUT THE AUTHOR

Dr Sophie Farooque is one of the UK's leading allergy experts. She is a Fellow of the Royal College of Physicians and was elected onto the council of the British Society of Allergy and Clinical Immunology in 2018. She is a practising NHS consultant at St Mary's Hospital in Paddington, and has been involved extensively in the UK's response following reports of COVID-19 vaccine allergy. She speaks regularly at medical conferences both nationally and abroad and has been quoted in the *Guardian* and *The Times,* among other news outlets. She has appeared on *This Morning,* Sky News and *The One Show.* She is passionate about empowering both healthcare professionals and patients to have confidence in managing allergy. Find her on Twitter: @LondonAllergy.

T0015392

PENGUIN LIFE EXPERTS SERIES

The Penguin Life Experts series equips readers with simple but vital information on common health issues and empowers readers to get to know their own bodies to better improve their health. Books in the series include:

Managing Your Migraine
by Dr Katy Munro

*****

Preparing for the Perimenopause and Menopause
by Dr Louise Newson

*****

Keeping Your Heart Healthy
by Dr Boon Lim

*****

Understanding Allergy
by Dr Sophie Farooque

*****

Managing IBS
by Dr Lisa Das

Next in the series, publishing in 2022:

*****

Living with ME and CFS
by Dr Gerald Coakley and Beverly Knops

Understanding Allergy

DR SOPHIE FAROOQUE

PENGUIN LIFE

AN IMPRINT OF

PENGUIN BOOKS

PENGUIN LIFE

UK | USA | Canada | Ireland | Australia
India | New Zealand | South Africa

Penguin Life is part of the Penguin Random House group of companies
whose addresses can be found at global.penguinrandomhouse.com.

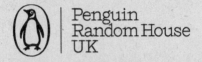

Penguin
Random House
UK

003

First published 2022

Copyright © Dr Sophie Farooque, 2022

The moral right of the author has been asserted

Set in 11.8/14.75pt Garamond MT Std
Typeset by Jouve (UK), Milton Keynes
Printed and bound in Great Britain by Clays Ltd, Elcograf S.p.A.

The authorized representative in the EEA is Penguin Random House Ireland,
Morrison Chambers, 32 Nassau Street, Dublin D02 YH68

A CIP catalogue record for this book is available from the British Library

ISBN: 978-0-241-52788-7

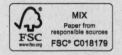

To my mother and father, to whom I owe everything.

Contents

Introduction

You might be picking up this book because you have an allergy, but even if you don't, the chances are that you will know someone who does.

Allergies have been rising at an astonishing rate in the industrial world and 44 per cent of British adults now report suffering from at least one allergy.[1] The majority of allergic disease starts in childhood, so children – and by extension their families – are not spared either. Put simply, the UK has never been more allergic, and more of us are itching, wheezing and sneezing our way through life than ever before.

Looking further afield, allergies are the most common chronic disease across Europe, with predictions that by 2025 half of all Europeans will be affected.[2] Fifty million Americans are reported to have an allergic disease, including 5.6 million children with food allergies,[3] and hospital admissions for life-threatening allergic reactions have increased fourfold in the past twenty years in Australia.[4] Across the globe, sales of 'free from' foods are soaring and prescriptions for adrenaline autoinjectors are rocketing. Tragic cases of anaphylaxis – a severe allergic reaction (see page 117) – appear in the headlines every few months. While these cases increase public awareness, they also provoke fear. Food allergy may not be the leading cause of death in people with food allergies (a statistical truth), but nobody wants to be that tragic headline.

Why Dr Google won't have the answers

With so many of us suffering, it is unsurprising that we search online for 'allergy' more frequently than 'migraine', 'heart attacks' and 'breast cancer'. Yet accessing specialist help, despite the increase in allergic disease, is not always easy.

Social-media feeds will often contain medical advice of varying quality, with hundreds of Facebook pages on allergy alone. Typing the question 'Am I allergic to . . . ?' into Google returns an incredible 51,000 results, and within this 'infodemic' are confusing, misleading and potentially harmful pages, as well as helpful results. In the spring and summer, searches for 'hay fever' overtake searches for 'allergy' itself.

At the same time, many family doctors and hospital specialists have had little formal allergy training, and there are few specialists in most countries, including the UK. Thus there is this huge mismatch between the numbers of people with allergic diseases and the specialist help available to support them. England didn't even have an allergy-specialist training programme until 2001, when I became the first doctor in the UK to enrol in the rigorous five-year specialist training programme. After completing it and a PhD, I found myself leading the oldest – and one of the largest – allergy services in the UK at St Mary's Hospital in London.

The clinic first became famous in the 1900s as the home of allergen immunotherapy, and in 1958 a remarkable doctor, Dr Bill Frankland, became its director. Widely known as the 'grandfather of allergy', he worked there until he retired in 1977. An allergist to the core, he was a founding member of the

British Society for Allergy & Clinical Immunology (BSACI) and was its president from 1963 to 1966. He transformed the lives of millions of hay-fever sufferers by being the first doctor to make the pollen count available to the general public and press (the meter lived on the roof of the hospital nurses' home). I met him in my first year of specialist training and he became both my friend and mentor. Ever curious and always asking questions, he used to attend medical conferences until a year or two before his death, aged 108. Filled with a love for people and especially his patients, Bill died in 2020 and a light from the allergy world was extinguished for ever.

Bill frequently commented to me that by the time patients saw him, they had suffered unnecessarily for years. Decades later, not much has changed. Stoicism, and a fatalism that nothing can be done, means that patients continue to present their symptoms to specialists late, often after many years of struggling. From runny noses, itchy eyes and miserable summers, to unexplained allergic reactions or multiple food allergies, I find there are few patients who do not benefit from specialist input. More than ever, the ability to transform a patient's life, sometimes in the space of just one visit, is one of the reasons I love my work as an allergist.

Perhaps more surprising, however, is that around half of the patients who come to my clinic are not allergic at all. And when it comes to drug allergy, the percentage who believe they might be allergic to a drug, but turn out not to be, is even higher, at around 90 per cent.

One case that sticks in the mind is of a lady who had been told she was allergic to local anaesthetic. Unable to find a dentist to treat her when she developed toothache, she ended up having the offending teeth extracted under general anaesthetic. On investigation in the drug-allergy clinic, it turned out that she had never been allergic to local anaesthetic and if we had seen her sooner, her teeth could have been saved.

Thankfully, not all cases are so dramatic, but all too often I see patients who have cut out foods from their diet, avoided a certain medication for years or ripped up their carpets to reduce levels of house dust mite – all in the mistaken belief that they are allergic. The situation is further complicated by allergy or intolerance tests being sold (often online) that frequently do not work. Patients part with their money for these tests and come to my clinic, only to be told that the test has no scientific validity. Even in cases where patients have proper allergy testing, the results are often misinterpreted. Allergy skin-prick and blood tests are an essential part of allergy diagnosis, but they only have value when taken in conjunction with an accurate and detailed allergy history.

Allergies can be tricky to diagnose, and often symptoms overlap with other medical conditions. So I began to organize study days to try and educate healthcare professionals, and increasingly I found myself being invited to speak at medical conferences in the UK and abroad. In 2016 I joined Twitter, one of my goals being to educate medical colleagues who were firefighting on the front lines. What is strikingly apparent is that an allergy label is all too easy to acquire, but far more difficult to remove.

During the COVID-19 pandemic, allergy again began to hit the headlines, with reports of allergic reactions to COVID-19 vaccines. We now know that allergic reactions to the vaccine are extremely rare, but even today allergists continue to allay concerns, to ensure that all eligible people are vaccinated and the unfounded fear of vaccination-related allergy is diminished.

How understanding allergy can help you and your family

A book felt like a natural next step for me: a book to help patients make sense of it all and to broaden awareness of allergies. In these pages I explain what allergies are and why we think they are increasing; their diagnosis and treatment; and you will also find tips on how to discuss allergies with your doctor, plus lots of myth-busting as we go along. There will be case histories too, but all the patient stories are published either with consent or anonymized.

The motto of the A&E department in my hospital is *Scientia vincet timorem* ('Knowledge conquers fear'). I believe this applies to many situations in life, and I would like this book to live up to that maxim. I want people to feel confident about managing their allergies, and also their families and friends to feel empowered to support them. All the recommendations in this book are based on scientific evidence and expert consensus.

You will find individual chapters on hay fever, food allergies, drug allergies and anaphylaxis. Allergies may group together in such a way that the same person will have more than one allergic condition. This book will enable you to look at allergies as a 'whole'. I will talk you through how to try and prevent allergies developing and will specifically discuss the relationship between eczema and food allergy. Towards the end of the book you will find two detailed appendices on how to avoid individual food allergens and questions to ask your doctor, as well as an extensive list of resources.

You can read this book in the order it is written or dip in and out, as takes your fancy. While acknowledging that it can never offer a substitute for medical advice, I wanted to create a credible resource, so that people could make decisions about their health with the most accurate information. *Understanding Allergy* is the definitive guide to allergic disease, and I hope reading it will change your life for the better.

1. What Are Allergies and Why Do They Matter?

'Allergy' is an umbrella term for a range of conditions. Some allergies are very common, such as hay fever, while others are extremely rare, such as exercise-induced anaphylaxis. In fact allergy is probably the only medical speciality where there is a high chance that the specialist you are seeing has the same condition!

Yet although allergy causes personal misery for millions of people globally, we are not always very good at treating it. In my experience this is for three main reasons: sufferers think there is nothing that can be done to help them; knowledge among healthcare professionals is lacking; and specialist clinics can be hard to access. It is estimated that up to 90 per cent of people living with allergy in the European Union are undertreated[1] or even untreated. Allergies are estimated to cost the NHS about £1 billion per year.[2] And despite so many of us suffering from them, the word 'allergy' is often misunderstood, because many conditions that can be allergy-related may also not be – for example, rhinitis (inflammation of the lining of the nose), eczema, asthma and even outbreaks of hives (red, itchy welts on the skin that can look like insect bites).

This lack of clarity has a knock-on effect. Many people worry unnecessarily about having an allergy when they do not have one. Patients who are allergic can have a different frustration, often reporting that because the word 'allergy' is overused, they struggle to be taken seriously.

Before we get to how to diagnose and find the right treatment for your allergies, let me take you through some of the basics. I want you to understand what allergies are and what is going on in your body. I often find that when my patients understand more about their allergy, they feel confident to deal with them and generally happier.

Allergy 101

Allergies occur when your body's defence – the immune system – views a substance as harmful and therefore reacts to it. An **allergen** is the medical term for the usually harmless substance, such as pollen or a food, that your immune system is now treating as rogue. Your immune system is highly developed and very effective at protecting the body from outside invaders, such as viruses, bacteria and parasites. When it works well, it keeps you safe and you barely notice it. But in the case of allergy, it has made a mistake and gone into overdrive. Instead of realizing that peanuts, dust or milk are completely harmless and should be ignored, the immune system treats them like an invader and responds. And it is this very specific immune response that can potentially be harmful.

> **What are food intolerances and sensitivities?**
> **Food intolerances are more common than allergy**
> **and refer to a reaction that doesn't involve the**
> **immune system. The problem is digestion.**
> **Intolerance to the milk-sugar lactose is very**

common. People don't have enough of the enzyme called lactase to break it down in their gut and, as a result, when they drink cow's milk or eat foods high in lactose, it can't be digested and they can develop an upset stomach, diarrhoea and bloating. If you are lactose-intolerant you can often have some dairy foods, but just not too much, which is not the case if you are allergic to milk (as here even a drop can trigger a severe reaction). Food intolerances can be unpleasant, but they are rarely dangerous.

Food sensitivity does not have a concrete medical definition, but is a loose term used to describe symptoms such as headaches, aches, tiredness and 'brain fog', and we don't really know what it means. Some patients feel their symptoms are triggered by multiple foods and hope to find a single test that will tell them exactly which foods to avoid so that they can feel better. Unfortunately, no scientifically proven test exists – despite a number of tests available online claiming to do so.

When allergies strike

We can develop an allergy at any time in our lives. Food allergies, hay fever and allergic asthma tend to develop earlier in life, while allergies to venom and medicines are more likely to develop as we get older. This probably reflects when we are exposed to these potential allergens. We encounter food and pollens from infancy, and usually encounter medicines and bee and wasp stings later in life.

Of course things do not always fit neatly into boxes. A recent study from the US found that a surprising number of adults were reporting convincing new food allergies, especially to shellfish.[3] Yet it still remains unusual to develop a new food allergy, or hay fever in middle age or later. Rather, if you develop one allergy in early childhood, you will often develop another along the way. Atopic dermatitis (eczema), food allergy, asthma and rhinitis will often cluster together in the same individual. This genetic tendency to develop allergy is called atopy and the treatment of one condition often influences the other.

So what is happening during an allergic reaction? To better understand, let's briefly step into the fascinating world of the immune system.

Border patrol

Your body is constantly defending itself from threats, but most of the time you are unaware of it. As you are reading this, you are blinking and this allows lubricating tears to spread out in a film across your eyes. Blinking physically protects your eyes from dust and irritating substances. Those tears don't just lubricate, but contain the natural antibiotic lysozyme, which kills bacteria. Then there's the nose – the ultimate air conditioner. Each day it filters out debris and warms and humidifies 10,000 litres (17,600 pints) of air. Mucus secreted by the cells lining your nostrils traps pathogens (microorganisms such as bacteria, viruses and parasites that can cause disease) before they enter the lungs. All the while your skin is acting as a physical barrier against bacteria and viruses, and your stomach will have been releasing acid to help with digestion and kill bacteria in your food.

Yet none of these actions involve your immune system. It is only if pathogens pass this first line of defence and 'breach security' that your immune system will get involved. Think of your immune system as an army that is on permanent border-patrol. Its soldiers are called white blood cells (WBCs) or leukocytes.

WBCs help safeguard your body against infection and disease. We each have about two trillion of them. They travel around your body, always on the lookout for danger. And just as there are lots of regiments in the army, so there are lots of different types of leukocytes in the immune-system army: T-cells, B-cells, dendritic cells, mast cells, basophils, neutrophils and macrophages, to name just a few, and they all do different things.

What happens during an allergic reaction?

Let's take food allergy as an example. Normally when a food is in your gut, it is sampled by numerous good bacteria. These have been present since you were born and have a multitude of important functions, including strengthening your gut barrier, teaching your immune system to recognize whether or not food is a threat and manufacturing vitamins. These good bacteria are so important that human breast milk contains complex sugars to feed one of the major bacterial players in our gut, called bifidobacteria. These sugars are indigestible by the baby; they are there to specifically feed the bifidobacteria.

Dendritic cells are WBCs and are the sentinels of your immune-system army. They are found all over your body. Usually they sit there and, like wine-tasters, sample the fluid around them; if there is nothing interesting, they spit it out. When dendritic cells are instructed by good bacteria, they will not be interested in food molecules passing through your gut barrier. They will inform the other leukocytes that everything is okay. We now have a situation of **immune tolerance**.

When your gut lacks good bacteria, your immune system lacks training, and allergies can occur because lots of WBCs are being activated that shouldn't be. The first stage in this process is called **sensitization** and this simply means that you have produced immunoglobulin E (IgE) allergy antibodies. Antibodies recognize invaders and help neutralize them, but peanut or pollen, for example, should not need neutralizing; and once you have IgE antibodies to a substance, some people (but not all) will develop an allergy.

Like your brain, your immune system has a form of memory. Let's take peanut as an example: once the immune system has produced peanut antibodies and identified peanut as a threat, it will keep on doing so, unless you are lucky enough to outgrow the allergy. This is why if you have an allergy, every time you are exposed to an allergen it will trigger a reaction known as an **allergic response**. Although your symptoms may vary (your hay fever may be worse one year than another, for example), they will occur every time that you are exposed to enough allergen.

Bacteria rule the world

So a food allergy is not just due to your DNA or bad luck: the bacteria in your gut are important and there is a complex immune process at play. And this extends beyond food allergy. A 2021 study found

that bacteria in the gut of adults with hay fever and allergic rhinitis had less diversity and different groups of bacteria dominated, compared to non-allergic individuals.[4] Allergists also suspect that whether an individual outgrows their allergy may be related to the balance of bacteria in the gut, but we can't be certain.

1. As you eat peanut, instead of spitting the peanut particles out, the dendritic cells 'swallow' them and become activated. They then travel to the lymph nodes, where the T-cells like to hang out. This is the moment your dendritic cell has been waiting for.

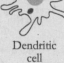

Peanut   Allergen   Dendritic cell

2. Once in the lymph node, the dendritic cell can now 'show and tell' the peanut it is proudly displaying to thousands of 'virgin' T-cells. These are T-cells that have never been activated and it will meet hundreds of them an hour. Once the dendritic cell finds a 'virgin' T-cell that can be activated specifically by peanut, and both cells 'agree' peanut is a danger, the peanut-specific T-cell transforms into a T-helper-2 cell (Th2 cell).

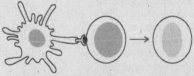

Dendritic cell   Peanut-specific T-cell   Th2 cell

3. The T-helper-2 cell informs the factory workers of your immune defence (the B-cells) by releasing chemicals called interleukins, which they need to start producing weapons to fight the intruder. These weapons are called antibodies.

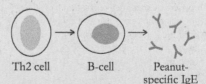

Th2 cell   B-cell   Peanut-specific IgE

4. The specific IgE to peanut produced by the B-cells sticks to receptors on the mast cell. You are now sensitized to peanut and are at risk of developing a peanut allergy.

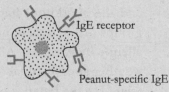

The peanut-specific IgE binds to the mast cell. They are now armed and ready to react

5. During an allergic reaction you eat peanut

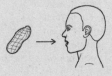

6. The peanut allergen is absorbed

7. This binds to your mast cells, which are covered in peanut-specific IgE. Mast cells live their lives waiting to explode. The peanut allergen fits like a 'key in a lock' and activates them. The mast cell then 'detonates' releasing histamine and other pre-packaged inflammatory chemicals.

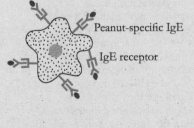

8. Thus symptoms we associate with allergy, such as itching, sneezing, congestion, wheezing and low blood pressure, may begin. One specific enzyme released by mast cells into the blood is called tryptase and this is often measured to confirm the diagnosis of a severe allergic reaction.

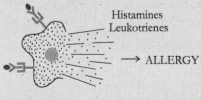

From sensitization to peanut allergy

Allergy v. sensitization

As we now know, allergy cannot develop without sensitization. However, there are some people who produce IgE against an allergen but don't get symptoms when they are re-exposed. For example, they have specific IgE to cat, but don't react when they come near a cat; or they have specific IgE to grass pollen, but don't get hay fever. And there are others who outgrow their allergy but their specific IgE remains. For example, they were allergic to egg as a very young child but could consume it freely once they reached primary school, yet their allergy tests remain positive. So why is this? The truth is that we don't know why some people stop at sensitization and others progress to allergy, nor do we really understand why some people who were allergic when younger may lose their allergy as they grow older.

All of this has one **very** important implication for you. If you have a positive allergy test, it does not automatically mean you are allergic. It simply means that your body has encountered an allergen and produced specific IgE against it. That is why an accurate diagnosis of allergy requires both a test and a consultation with a doctor who understands how these tests work. Your detailed allergy history is the bridge between your allergy-test results and being diagnosed with an allergy. Using allergy tests to 'screen' for allergy is not what they were designed for and should be avoided (see page 79).

Mast cells: the mischief-makers

Mast cells are made in the bone marrow and are found in our tissues and live for months. Normally they play a protective role in fighting pathogens and help regulate our immune response, but as you have learned, they can also be activated by allergies and cause all sorts of mischief. As well as releasing histamine and other inflammatory chemicals, once they are activated they can synthesize other molecules that will tell other white blood cells that they need to join the battle. Too many mast cells, or overactive mast cells, can lead to conditions such as mastocytosis and mast cell activation syndrome, but these rare illnesses are beyond the scope of this book.

Are all allergic reactions due to IgE?

No, allergic reactions can be IgE-mediated or non-IgE-mediated. The vast majority of allergic reactions are mediated by IgE antibodies. These reactions usually occur very rapidly and will be my main focus in this book.

More rarely reactions can be non-IgE-mediated and are due to cell reactions within the immune system. Delayed cow's milk protein allergy (CMPA) falls into this category. Many drug allergies can also be non-IgE-mediated, such as allergies to aspirin, paracetamol and certain antibiotics (see Chapter 11). We suspect that almost all allergic reactions to the COVID-19 vaccines fall into this group, too (see Chapter 5). Contact allergies, for example, to hair dye or nickel are also non-IgE mediated and are due to our T-cells misbehaving.

This is important because if there is no specific IgE, then allergy skin-prick tests and conventional allergy blood tests become completely useless. For example, the only way to confirm or exclude a non-IgE-mediated drug allergy is for the patient to try the drug again. This is called a drug challenge, and I run regular clinics where patients are given a medication again, under careful allergy-specialist supervision. In the case of non-IgE-mediated food allergy (see Chapter 8) there are different approaches, but again skin-prick testing is not usually helpful, while in the case of contact allergies, patch-testing is used. Patch-testing involves sticking tiny amounts of contact allergens to the skin on your back using a special tape. After forty-eight hours the patches are removed and your skin is checked to see if there has been any reaction. Contact allergies are not associated with allergy. Thousands of substances can cause a reaction and the commonest are rubber chemicals, preservatives, metals, perfumes, cosmetics and plants. Patch-testing is a specialist field in itself, and in the UK clinics are run by skin specialists. It's a fascinating area, but further discussion lies outside the scope of this book.

So now that you have a basic understanding of the principles, let's continue our journey and delve into the intriguing world of allergic disease.

2. The Allergy Epidemic

There was a boy in my class at school called Philip who was known for two things: hay fever and being the only one among us who owned a Sony Discman. His fame was seasonal: hay fever dominated the summer stories, and the Discman dominated the rest of the year. Philip was a good runner, but every summer the joke went that his nose did more running than he did. By the time I left school, Philip was no longer quite as unique: not only did more of us possess a Discman and had developed hay fever, but someone a few years below had joined the club with a food allergy.

At that time I was wholly unaware that the increase in allergies I was witnessing among my classmates was part of the steep rise in allergic disease. In the last thirty to forty years allergies have become a major public-health issue across the UK, Europe, North America and Australasia. Initially there was an increase in the number of people suffering from rhinitis and asthma. This was followed by a second wave, as food allergies surged.

In addition South Africa has one of the highest prevalence rates of allergic disorders in the developing world and is fast catching up on the US, New Zealand, Australia and Europe. And an increasing prevalence of allergic rhinitis and asthma has been reported in the Indian subcontinent.

To put this into context: mentions of allergic rhinitis can be found in Islamic texts in the ninth century and in sixteenth-century European texts; however, hay fever was only first described in any detail in the nineteenth century (see Chapter 3), when it was regarded as a highly unusual, rare condition.[1] Yet the numbers of us affected have gradually climbed: nowadays we will all know someone who itches, sneezes and wheezes through the pollen season.

And before the 1990s peanut allergy was so rare that barely any data was collected, but since then more than 3,000 scientific papers on the topic have been published. Food allergies are so common that most schools across the land will have one or two children in each class who have been diagnosed with one. In the UK there was an average 5.7 per cent year-on-year increase in the number of people admitted to hospital with allergic reactions to food between 1998 and 2008.

> **In numbers: the modern global allergy epidemic**
> So where are we now? Let's look at the stats.
> - The UK has one of the highest incidences of allergy in the world.[2]
> - The European Academy of Allergy and Clinical Immunology (EAACI) estimates that by 2025 about half the population of the EU will be affected by at least one type of allergy.[3]
> - More than fifty million Americans suffer from allergies each year, costing in excess of US $18 billion per annum.[4]
> - 10 per cent of Australian children under one year of age have a proven food allergy.[5]
> - Asthma affects one in seven adolescents and young adults in Europe.

- **Allergic rhinitis affects around one in four thirteen-to fourteen-year-olds in India.**[6]
- **Hay fever affects up to 30 per cent of the population in parts of China.**[7]
- **The UK has seen a 336 per cent increase in the number of adrenaline autoinjectors (AAIs) prescribed between 1998 and 2018.**[8]

Currently data remains slanted towards the Anglosphere and Europe, and the situation in countries such as Brazil, India and parts of Africa where there is limited access to testing and research funding is less clear, particularly when it comes to food allergies.

However, while the extent of the rise in allergies is debated amongst specialists, nobody can deny that the number of people affected globally has really increased. In 2003 a Royal College of Physicians report described the rise in allergic disease in the UK as an epidemic and called for allergy services to be expanded.

In this chapter I will look at the latest evidence and thinking behind the allergy epidemic. This is a rapidly evolving area and, as allergists, we are only starting to scratch the surface. If I were to update this book in ten years' time, this chapter would probably change the most.

Let's break it down into layers.

Layer 1: the genetic risk of allergy

We know that our genes influence our susceptibility to develop allergic disease, but this is also influenced by our environment. For example, a South-East Asian child born in Australia has around a 1,400 per cent increased risk of developing a food allergy, compared to their counterparts born in Singapore, despite similar genetics.[9] Another study carried out in Birmingham, the UK's second-largest city, found that children of Indian, Pakistani and Bangladeshi heritage were at higher risk of severe anaphylaxis compared to white British children.[10] Canadian-born children of South-East and East Asian parents versus all other ethnicities reported more food allergy.[11] These three studies – and many others – highlight the importance of the interplay between our genes and our environment (this is called epigenetics). Broadly speaking, if you have one parent with an allergy, you have a 30–50 per cent of risk of developing an allergy yourself. If both parents have an allergy, this rises to 60–80 per cent.

Layer 2: the microbiome, our invisible organ

As we develop in the womb, we are cocooned in a sterile environment of amniotic fluid. Our first exposure to bacteria comes at birth, as we travel through the birth canal, where we pick up our very own starter pack of bacteria from our mother and begin developing our own microbiota.

The microbiota is the sum of all the microorganisms that live both in and on our body, and they outnumber us. The average 70-kg (11-stone) man is made up of thirty trillion human cells and a community of forty trillion vitally important bacteria, fungi and viruses. The term microbiome is often used interchangeably with the word microbiota, but technically refers to the genetic material of all the microbes living within us.

Try thinking of the microbiota as an invisible organ of the body. It weighs around 1.36kg (3lb) and helps us out in all sorts of ways. It assists in the digestion of food, protects us from harmful bacteria, regulates our immune system and manufactures vitamins B_{12} and K. Our gut microbiota changes quickly in early childhood and stabilizes by the time we are about three years old. However, it is not static and will change throughout our lives, with diet, stress levels and medication all shaping it as we age. (*Managing IBS* by leading gastroenterologist Dr Lisa Das is another book in the Penguin Life Expert series that covers the microbiome in fascinating detail.)

How does the microbiome link to allergy?

We strongly suspect that being exposed to a range of bacterial products in early life makes the developing immune system much calmer and more well behaved. Think of your gut as a finishing school, packed full of bacteria ready to teach your immune system how to direct itself properly. The aim is to educate your immune system to recognize and be ready to fight an infection, but if that interaction goes wrong (probably due to the balance and types of bacteria), then we seem to become more susceptible to allergy.

A 2020 South African study of children assessed allergy risk factors in urban and rural settings. It found that exposure to farm animals in infants and their mothers during pregnancy was protective against allergic outcomes for rural children, compared to an increased risk of food allergy for urban children and those delivered via Caesarean section. However, for these children consumption of fermented milk products reduced the risk of asthma and eczema.[12] In the UK babies living in a home with a dog are less likely to develop a food allergy.[13] An international 2014 study of 500,000 children reinforced previous research, showing that large families and younger children are less likely to develop hay fever or eczema. The 'sibling effect' is linked to increased exposure to germs, making the younger child's microbiota more diverse and healthy.[14]

There are various factors affecting whether bacteria that protect against allergy build up in the gut:

- **Antibiotics**: Numerous studies have found an association between exposure to antibiotics and the risk of childhood allergy. A Japanese study of more than 1,000 children found that taking antibiotics in the first two years of life increased the likelihood of children developing asthma, eczema and allergic rhinitis by the time they reached five.[15] Australian researchers reviewed the health records of more than 30,000 children, finding that the prescription of three or more antibiotics was associated with food allergy and rhinitis, especially in younger children.[16] In a European study of 1,080 children, exposure to antibiotics during pregnancy was associated with a 1.6-times increased risk of eczema and a three-times increased risk of food allergy in infants.[17]

- **Caesarean section**: Babies born by Caesarean section will be exposed to different bacteria and will develop a different microbiota from those born vaginally. A large number of (but not all) studies have shown that birth by Caesarean section is linked to allergic disease, and children may be at higher risk of developing asthma-type symptoms.[18] Assisted birth and vacuum delivery have also been associated with an allergic predisposition,[19] and it is thought that again this may be due to changes in the composition of the microbiome.

- **Dummies**: Perhaps one of the clearest suggestions that a skewed microbiome can increase the chance of developing an allergy came from a study published in 2021. Almost 900 Australian infants were studied. Researchers found that if a baby's dummy was repeatedly cleaned with antiseptic agents during the first six months of life there was an increased risk of food allergy. If antiseptic was not used, there was no increased risk. This increase was presumably due to the chemicals in the antiseptic disrupting the microbiome in the baby's mouth and gut.[20]

Layer 3: the dual-allergen exposure hypothesis

One weekend while I was working in the laboratory and researching my PhD I bumped into a fellow medical trainee specializing in children's allergy, called Helen Brough. Now an eminent paediatric allergist, at that time she was also reading for a PhD and, in a testament to the unglamorous nature of research, was spending her time vacuuming living-room floors and children's mattresses and analysing the dust collected for peanut protein. A long conversation followed and two things resulted: the first was a wonderful friendship, and the second was that I heard for the first time about the dual-allergen exposure hypothesis.

Helen explained that she was researching how easily peanut allergen could spread in our houses after eating, and whether it could be removed easily. She had found that if you ate a peanut-butter sandwich in your home, remarkably by the following day peanut allergen had spread throughout your house. The peanut allergen was measurable on hands and in saliva even three hours after consuming peanuts, allowing peanut to spread for many hours. Peanut dust was found in children's beds and even 60°C (140°F) washing of the bedding only reduced, rather than eliminated, peanut protein levels. So even if they were not eating peanut directly, many young children were having environmental exposure to peanut at home.[21]

She commented that there was an increasing body of evidence suggesting that exposure to food allergens via the skin in early life could increase a child's chance of developing a food allergy – an allergic response might literally be skin-deep. However, if those same allergenic foods were introduced into the diet from an early age, it could be protective. This was highlighted in a 2003 study, in which a staggering 91 per cent of infants with confirmed peanut allergy had creams containing peanut oil rubbed onto their skin in their first six months of life.[22] Researchers believed this was why infants with eczema were particularly vulnerable to developing a food allergy. And this didn't only apply to foods – eczema in childhood was also associated with a doubling of risk of developing asthma and hay fever.

Layer 4: vitamin D

Like many areas in this whole field, it is suspected (but not proven) that vitamin D (sometimes called the 'sunshine vitamin') may be important in regulating the microbiota in the gut. Therefore we may be suffering higher allergy rates because we are spending more and more time indoors and are practising sun-safe behaviours. The evidence is not as strong as with other areas of research, but there is some evidence to suggest that vitamin D deficiency is associated with an increased risk of atopy, asthma and food allergy. However, it is too early to say whether Vitamin D supplementation can reduce or even reverse allergy.

So we can see that it is apparent there is no one single reason driving the rise in allergies, and that external environmental factors and internal factors from within our bodies are fuelling the allergy epidemic. The microbiome in particular is critical. Its most important task is to educate and train our immune system. This means that we need the right microbes, at the right time and in the right place, and if there is an imbalance then our risk of developing allergy increases. We still have a lot to learn and we are still missing pieces of the puzzle, but we have reached the point where an increased understanding of the reasons for the rise is giving way to simple steps that we can take to try and prevent allergic disease (see Chapter 14).

3. Runny Nose and Itchy Eyes: Understanding Hay Fever and Rhinitis

I had just started training in allergy when the opportunity arose to attend a three-day national conference. It was a big deal: the cream of the UK allergy world would be there, and I wanted to make a good impression. During the opening session my nose began to itch and run. I tried to suppress it, but a series of very loud sneezes reverberated through the lecture theatre. So loud that half the attendees turned to try and locate where the noise was coming from, and the speaker joked that 'Someone couldn't leave their allergies at home.'

I dashed out during the break to buy some tissues, convinced that my symptoms must be psychosomatic. I mean, who wouldn't have an itchy nose at an allergy conference? Yet my symptoms continued after I got home, and it slowly dawned on me that perhaps for the first time in my life I had developed an allergy.

As it was early summer, my immediate thought was hay fever. When I returned to work, I got myself skin-tested to grass pollen, but my skin-prick test was negative. I was baffled. Two days later I repeated the skin test. Again negative. One evening after clinic I decided to test myself for another likely cause of these symptoms – house dust mite (HDM). Within ten minutes I felt an itch on my arm. I looked down and there was a large, juicy wheal at the site of my skin test. I had joined the estimated 26 per cent of UK adults who suffer from allergic rhinitis.[1]

Allergic rhinitis is one of the most common medical conditions for which help is sought. The prevalence ranges from 11.8 per cent in Oviedo (Spain) to 46 per cent in Melbourne (Australia).[2] Often people who have allergic rhinitis will also have asthma, and how well one is controlled impacts the other. In this chapter we will look at the causes and telltale symptoms of allergic rhinitis to get to the bottom of the sneezing, runny noses and streaming eyes that so many of us know and loathe, before moving on to the main culprit allergens themselves (pollens, cats and HDM). Look out for the pollen calendar on page 35 if you think pollen is triggering your symptoms.

What rhinitis is – and why the term 'hay fever' is misleading

In Greek *rhin* means 'nose' and *itis* means 'inflammation', so rhinitis is inflammation of the nose.

The most common trigger for rhinitis is infection, usually due to a cold. And once infections are excluded, rhinitis can be divided into allergic and non-allergic types. Making that distinction is crucial in working out how to keep symptoms at bay. If you are allergic, then allergen avoidance may be helpful; but if you are not, it will make no difference.

I will briefly discuss non-allergic rhinitis later (see page 30), but for now let's focus on allergic rhinitis – that is, inflammation of the inside of the nose caused by an allergen, such as pollen or an animal.

Allergic rhinitis is often classified as being either seasonal or perennial (where symptoms persist all year round). The common term for seasonal allergic rhinitis is hay fever – a misnomer originating in nineteenth-century England. In an early example of 'fake news', the spurious idea that the smell of fresh hay triggered symptoms spread rapidly across the continent, and to this day seasonal allergic rhinitis remains known as hay fever throughout Europe. The Norwegians can be credited for being marginally more accurate, dropping the term 'fever' for 'cold', so if you are Norwegian you have a 'hay cold' instead. The bottom line: hay is not responsible for seasonal symptoms and there is no fever.

This seasonal-versus-perennial split works well in countries like the UK with defined pollen seasons, but less so in countries where the seasons are less clear-cut. So another classification that is widely used is intermittent-versus-persistent:[3]

- **Intermittent**: Where symptoms occur for fewer than four days a week and for fewer than four consecutive weeks.
- **Persistent**: Where symptoms occur for more than four days a week and for more than four consecutive weeks.

This classification is especially useful if someone is allergic to both seasonal and perennial allergens.

Key symptoms of allergic rhinitis

- Itchy nose, eyes, throat or inner ear
- Sneezing
- A runny nose
- Nasal blockage

With rhinitis, your nose is irritable, so you may find that strong smells like cigarette smoke, perfume and traffic fumes trigger symptoms.

Post-nasal drip, non-allergic rhinitis and one-sided nasal symptoms

Post-nasal drip is a tricky symptom, as you need to understand why it is occurring before treating it. Glands in our nose and throat constantly produce mucus and we all produce a couple of pints a day (estimates vary). This mucus cleans the nasal lining, traps and filters what is inhaled and moistens the air. We are usually unaware of swallowing it, but if the volume of mucus increases or it becomes thicker than usual, we notice it dripping down the back of our throat. People with post-nasal drip may report constantly having to clear their throat. Common causes include acid reflux, sinusitis with bacterial infection and vasomotor rhinitis (an overly sensitive nose). Treatments vary and may include sinus-rinsing, sprays to dry nasal secretions, or treating acid reflux or the sinus infection that is causing it. Post-nasal drip is almost never the dominant symptom in allergic rhinitis, but is more commonly seen in non-allergic rhinitis.

Patients with non-allergic rhinitis may also have a sneezy, congested, runny nose but, unlike an allergy, your immune system is not involved. Common causes of non-allergic rhinitis include:

1. Vasomotor rhinitis, where the nose is easily irritated, such as by smoke or fumes or changes in atmospheric temperature
2. Eosinophilic rhinitis: eosinophils are a WBC and can boost inflammation
3. Overuse of nasal decongestants
4. Hormonal changes, such as in pregnancy.

It can sometimes be difficult to distinguish between allergic and non-allergic rhinitis, which is why allergy testing can be helpful, but one useful clue is associated symptoms of itchy eyes, throat or nose. In non-allergic rhinitis this will not usually be present, because no histamine is being released.

Note: If your symptoms only affect one side of your nose, you probably don't have an allergy. Loss of smell, a thick green nasal discharge or crusting, and a nasal blockage without any other allergic-rhinitis symptoms are also unlikely to be due to an allergy. You should talk to a healthcare professional, who may refer you to an ear, nose and throat (ENT) specialist to exclude other conditions, such as chronic sinusitis and nasal polyps.

Counting the cost of rhinitis

Despite allergic rhinitis being the most common immunological disease in the world, I wasn't taught about it in medical school. Perhaps if it were renamed 'expensive rhinitis' it would have made it onto the curriculum.

- Rhinitis is costly: hay fever alone is said to be responsible for more than four million sick days worldwide and costs the British economy £300 million a year in lost productivity.
- Rhinitis affects both mental health and quality of life: one study suggests that adults with allergic and non-allergic rhinitis are 40 per cent more likely to develop depression.[4]
- Poorly controlled rhinitis can be dangerous: 7 per cent of people with allergic rhinitis report a car accident or near-miss because of uncontrolled symptoms, approximating to seven million accidents in the EU alone.[5]
- Global allergic rhinitis is estimated to cost $24.8 billion and asthma more than $90 billion.[6]

What causes seasonal allergic rhinitis?

Tree, grass and weed pollens are largely responsible for seasonal allergic rhinitis. The moulds *Alternaria* and *Cladosporium* can also trigger symptoms, but allergies to these are rarer.

Derived from the Greek word meaning 'fine flour', pollen is a powder that fertilizes plants. While flowers rely on insects to spread their pollen, as their pollen is too sticky and heavy to be airborne, trees, grasses and weeds rely on the wind to distribute their pollen from one plant to another. Plants that rely on wind pollination release light, powdery pollen that can be carried long distances by the wind. Massive quantities of pollen are often released: it is estimated that a single American ragweed plant can produce up to one billion pollen grains.

When we inhale this lighter airborne pollen, allergic symptoms are triggered.

What plants should I watch out for, and when?

In Europe early-flowering trees release their pollen in winter and spring and are responsible for allergic rhinitis in the first four months of the year. Hazel-tree pollen (*Corylus avellana*), plane-tree pollen (*Platanus acerifolia*) and silver-birch tree pollen (*Betula verrucosa*) are common culprits, while in warmer parts of the world, such as the Mediterranean and South Africa, olive (*Olea europea*) and cypress trees (*Cupressaceae* species) add their pollen into the mix. As trees stop pollinating, the grass season begins. Timothy grass (*Phleum pratense*) releases its pollen in May and June, with levels dropping off by mid-July in most European countries. From late summer to early autumn, weed pollen takes over, and mugwort (*Artemesia vulgaris*) is often a cause of symptoms. A similar pattern of hay fever is also seen in India, although the grass-pollen season runs later and is usually between September and December.[7]

In the US and Canada, ragweed (*Ambrosia artemisiifolia*) causes countless spoiled summers and will last until the first frost of the autumn. In the southern hemisphere, allergic rhinitis occurs from September to the end of December, with rye grass (*Lolium perenne*) and Bermuda grass (*Cynodon dactylon*) taking the top billing. In the Mediterranean and parts of Australia, pellitory (*Parietaria officinalis*) or the ominously nicknamed 'asthma weed' (*Parietaria judaica*) also triggers much itching, sneezing and wheezing. The word *Parietaria* derives from the Latin *paries*, meaning 'wall'. It is commonly found on roadsides and in gardens and thrives in cracks, especially against walls.

And it appears that, thanks to climate change, hay fever may affect even more of us in years to come. Described by scientists as 'Miracle-Gro for weeds', climate change is leading to increases in pollen concentrations, longer pollen seasons and different pollens triggering symptoms. Two papers published within one month in 2021 alone point to this concerning trend for patients and doctors alike. The first collected US data between 1990 and 2018 and found an almost three-week lengthening of the pollen season and a 21 per cent increase in pollen concentrations in that eighteen-year period.[8] The second study looked at the effect of climate change on pollen concentrations across north-west Europe: scientists discovered that a doubling of carbon-dioxide levels would translate into an increase in future grass-pollen allergy seasonal severity of up to 60 per cent.[9] Furthermore, as a result of global warming, ragweed, which was traditionally confined to the US, is increasingly causing symptoms of hay fever in France, northern Italy, Austria, Hungary[10] and other parts of Europe (affecting an estimated 15.8 million people).[11] And more extreme short-duration thunderstorms are likely in the future, with the associated risk of thunderstorm asthma (see page 40).

I think I might have allergic rhinitis – what should I do?

If your symptoms are mild and are well controlled with an antihistamine and/or a saline rinse (we will be going through

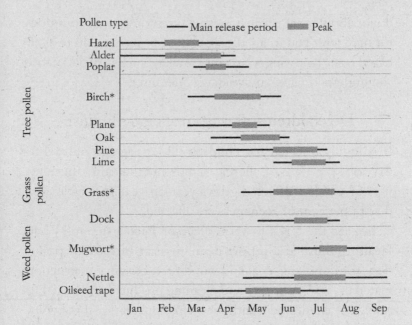

Pollen calendar

* These pollens tend to dominate the pollen calendar that is common to the UK and northern Europe. If you live in the Mediterranean, Australia or North America, check with your medical team or local allergy organizations for a pollen calendar where you live. For example, ragweed pollen will peak in mid-September in most parts of North America.

how to choose an antihistamine and other treatments in the next chapter) there is little else you need to do.

However, if your symptoms are disrupting your work or studies, affecting your sleep or making it hard to exercise, then you should talk to your family doctor, who can usually diagnose allergic rhinitis based on your symptoms, but will also pick up on any symptoms that are not typical. If there is a doubt about what is causing your symptoms, then your doctor may refer you to an allergy clinic for allergy skin tests or blood tests. Knowing what you are allergic to is crucial before you undertake allergen-avoidance measures.

Do children suffer from allergic rhinitis?

It is highly unusual for children under the age of two to develop symptoms of allergic rhinitis, but thereafter the numbers of children affected grows year-on-year. It is estimated that 15 per cent of teenagers are affected.

In 2020 the UK's Royal College of Paediatrics and Child Health published a report detailing that **indoor** air pollution from smoking, coal and wood fires, certain construction materials, aerosol sprays and cleaning products was linked to a range of childhood health problems, including asthma, rhinitis, conjunctivitis and eczema. It also observed that indoor air quality tended to relate closely to poor-quality housing. Solving this clearly involves change at a government level as well as from individuals, but some simple strategies that you can consider include banning smoking in the home, ventilating your kitchen during and after cooking and using chemical-free cleaning products.[12]

Poorly controlled allergic rhinitis can have a real impact on children and teenagers, from sports participation to academic performance: one study of 1,800 UK teenagers with allergic rhinitis symptoms found they were 40 per cent more likely to drop a grade between their mock and final exams. This rose to 70 per cent if they were taking a sedating antihistamine treatment.[13]

While it is straightforward to make a diagnosis of allergic rhinitis in adults and teenagers, it can be trickier in young children, as they frequently have colds and runny noses. Here are some signs to look out for:

1. If children are rubbing their eyes and itching their nose frequently, it could be an allergy. If they are clearly triggered each time they are exposed to an allergen, you can be fairly certain they have allergic rhinitis.
2. Our noses are anatomically and functionally linked to our eyes, sinuses, throat, middle ear, larynx and lower airway. If your child has chronic ear problems or glue ear, mouth-breathes and/or snores heavily, has a chronic cough or asthma that is hard to control, ask your family doctor if they think allergic rhinitis is a contributing factor.
3. The 'allergic salute' is a faint crease across the bridge of the nose, caused by constant rubbing. Your child may also display 'allergic shiners' – darkened discoloration below the eye, which is associated with nasal allergy.
4. Asthma and allergic rhinitis often go hand-in-hand, so if children have one, then they may also have the other, so raise this with your doctor.

If children have symptoms affecting one side of their nose only or are permanently blocked, they should be seen by an ENT surgeon. Allergic rhinitis symptoms are rare in the under-twos, so again this would be a cue for a referral to paediatric ENT.

The 'united airways theory'

Your respiratory tract starts in the nose and ends in the lungs – think of it as having the same paving (that is, the same cells) all the way down. So your nasal passages and airways are linked, both anatomically and immunologically, and inflammation in one part of the airways influences the other part. Therefore if an allergen causes inflammation in the nose, this inflammation can spread and affect the breathing tubes in your lungs, leading to asthma. This is known as the 'united airways theory'.

This is why pollen particles, which are usually too large to enter the lungs directly, can trigger a condition called seasonal asthma. This describes asthma that only strikes at certain times of the year, usually when the pollen count is high, and it implies an allergic cause. If you have never had a diagnosis of asthma, but experience classic asthma, symptoms such as wheezing, breathlessness and coughing along with hay fever, you could have seasonal asthma.

And rhinitis triggering asthma, or vice versa, is not just seasonal. Asthma and rhinitis are closely linked, with an estimated 80 per cent of people with asthma suffering from allergic rhinitis. So when I see patients with poorly controlled allergic rhinitis, I know it is highly likely that if they are asthmatic, then their asthma will be troublesome, too – and that all adds up to the emotional, physical and financial cost of managing both conditions.

Therefore if you have both allergic rhinitis and asthma, you need to keep both conditions under control using a two-pronged approach. We will talk more about managing allergic rhinitis in the next chapter, but the bottom line is that controlling your allergic rhinitis will usually reduce your symptoms of asthma.

If you do have asthma there are three important questions to ask yourself:

1. Do you have a personalized asthma-management plan?
2. Can you use your asthma inhalers effectively?
3. Do you have a yearly review with your family doctor?

If the answer to any of these questions is no, then please speak to your family doctor. This book does not cover the detailed diagnosis and management of allergic and non-allergic asthma, but asthma-management plans are often available for free online. Once completed, they will contain essential information to manage your asthma, and you can fill them in with your family doctor or the practice nurse.

If you have seasonal asthma, your doctor should prescribe you a regular preventer corticosteroid inhaler just prior to the start and continuing through the pollen season, to dampen down inflammation in the lower airways. In case of emergency your doctor will also prescribe you a rescue inhaler (usually blue in colour), to help to open up the airways by relaxing the small muscles that tighten them. If you remain symptomatic and/or are using your rescue inhaler at least three times per week, book another appointment with your doctor, as this suggests that your asthma (seasonal or otherwise) may not be under control and requires review and possible changes to your medication.

Thunderstorm asthma: an imperfect storm

Normally pollen is too large to enter your lungs, but when a thunderstorm is brewing, updraughts of air can lift whole pollen grains into the clouds. When exposed to moisture, these grains rupture into tiny pieces and this makes them highly allergenic. Windy downdraughts then carry these fragments to ground level, resulting in a 'pollen shower', and the minute fragments can be inhaled deep into your lungs, triggering an asthma attack. Grass pollens and moulds can be fragmented into allergenic particles, but tree pollen (even in fragments) does not usually cause thunderstorm asthma.

Thankfully, thunderstorm asthma is rare, but when it occurs it can be catastrophic. And it catches people out, as it can affect people with hay fever only. The largest known outbreak was in Melbourne in Australia in 2016, when paramedics responded to 1,900 emergency calls and, sadly, ten people died.[14] While Melbourne remains the epicentre of thunderstorm asthma, outbreaks have been described across the world, including in the UK, continental Europe and the US. However, the vast majority of thunderstorms will not trigger thunderstorm asthma, even when the pollen count is high. Nonetheless it is worth getting into the habit of checking the weather forecast and knowing what to do if a thunderstorm is predicted:

1. Remain indoors with the windows closed before and during the storm.
2. If you must go outside, wear a mask to avoid inhaling the pollen fragments.

3. If you have an asthma attack during a thunderstorm, take double-dose antihistamines.

4. Follow the four steps of asthma first aid, a useful process developed by Asthma Australia:[15] if you develop a sudden severe asthma attack, take four puffs of your reliever and wait four minutes. If there is no improvement, take another four puffs and wait another four minutes. If there is still no improvement, call for an ambulance and keep taking four separate puffs of your reliever inhaler every four minutes until help arrives.

Perennial allergic rhinitis

HDM and pets are the usual triggers of year-round symptoms (although in some countries cockroach saliva, faeces, eggs and shed skins are also highly relevant allergens), but before you rip out your carpets or start bathing your cat, let me tell you a little more about these common indoor allergens.

House dust mite (HDM)

With an average length of just 0.2–0.3mm, HDMs cause a big problem for such small creatures. They are the number-one cause of year-round rhinitis symptoms and allergic asthma.

There are two main species: the European house dust mite (*Dermatophagoides pteronyssinus*) and its American cousin (*Dermatophagoides farinae*). *Derma* means 'skin' and *phago* means 'to eat or devour'. Dead skin cells are the HDM's favourite meal. With most of us spending hours each night in bed, you can see why your bedding is a very attractive place for an

HDM to set up home, and why allergic individuals often say that their symptoms are worse when they wake up. For the record, HDMs are not the main constituent of household dust, which is mainly composed of clothing and carpet fibre, pet hair, pollen, dirt and sand.

Although HDMs are blind, they are light-sensitive and live deep within your pillows, mattresses and carpets. Their presence is not a marker of poor hygiene – HDMs are found in the fanciest bed sheets and mattresses. According to the American College of Allergy, Asthma and Immunology, 10 per cent of the weight of an old unwashed pillow will comprise dead HDMs and their droppings. They live for sixty-five to one hundred days and there are at least 100,000 dust mites in a foam mattress (spring mattresses contain lower numbers).[16] They reproduce sexually, with copulation lasting up to two days (!), the consequence of the mites' tiny size allowing only single-file exit of the sperm from the male. Each female will lay fifty to eighty eggs during her lifetime.[17]

HDMs have several unpleasant features that explain why they are so allergy-inducing. First, their droppings contain high concentrations of nasty allergens. And each mite produces about 1,000 droppings in its lifetime. Second, unfortunately these droppings easily become airborne when we are sweeping, vacuuming or changing bedding. And once they are in the air, we can easily breathe them in, worsening allergic rhinitis and asthma. In addition, killing dust mites isn't easy, and there is no way to get rid of a dust-mite colony completely. If food is limited, HDMs practice coprophagia, or eating their own faeces, as they are nutrient-rich and this prolongs their survival.[18] So when people talk about being allergic to HDM, they mean allergic to their faeces as well as the mites themselves.

However, HDMs do have one weakness: they don't drink water, but have to suck it out of the air. This means that they require at least 50 per cent humidity to survive. Remember this fact: it will be relevant when we discuss allergen avoidance and how to decrease their numbers in the next chapter.

Do dairy products give me a snotty nose?

The belief that 'milk causes mucus', and should be avoided when you have a cold or rhinitis, is something I often hear from patients.

While it is true that the proteins in milk and other dairy products will cause your saliva to become thicker and stickier and will make you feel as if you are producing more mucus, it will not increase the manufacture of mucus by your body.

The truth about cats and dogs

You might think you are allergic to cats or dogs because of their fur, but if you are reacting, you are allergic to proteins in their saliva, skin or urine. Cats are the allergen 'superspreaders' of the animal world, and at least eight allergenic proteins have been identified from them. The best known of these is the cat allergen Fel d1, a small, sticky protein secreted in cat saliva and its sebaceous and anal glands. When a cat grooms, it covers itself in saliva and, by extension, Fel d1. As the saliva dries, Fel d1 vaporizes and can stay airborne for days at a time. In addition, cat hairs that are shed will be covered in this sticky allergen. This, coupled with the fact that cats will explore every inch of the house and will rub up against their owners – covering them, their clothes and their shoes in allergen – means that cat allergen is literally everywhere.

Fel d1 is frequently measured in places where cats do not live, such as pubs, hotels, schools, cinemas and aeroplanes. This major cat allergen has also been detected in the Antarctic, although cats have never been there. It was even measured in dust from the NASA space shuttle! Therefore on the rare occasions my patients decide to rehome their cat because it is triggering allergy, I recommend a deep clean of carpeting, curtains and (if affordable) buying in completely new bedding.

Cat allergy is more common than dog allergy. Usually if an individual is allergic to one cat, they will react to most others. But when it comes to dog allergies, there are many people who are allergic to some breeds and not others. The only way to find out is if you are exposed to it. So if you are desperate for a dog, spend some time with the dog you have chosen, cuddle it and stroke it, and if you have no symptoms you will probably be okay. But if you kiss and cuddle the dog and develop an itchy, swollen face, or you start to sneeze or wheeze, then you should think about an alternative pet.

Myth-buster: is there such a thing as a hypoallergenic cat or dog?

You may have heard of 'hypoallergenic' cats and dogs – so named because they either shed less fur or have been bred to produce a lower quantity of the major cat and dog allergens in their dander. Unfortunately, decreased shedding of pet hair does not eliminate exposure to dog/cat saliva or to the other allergenic proteins to which an allergic person may have been sensitized.

Studies have shown no significant differences between levels of dog allergen in homes with hypoallergenic dogs compared to ordinary dogs.[19] Every cat or dog has saliva and skin and sebaceous glands. There is no animal that produces no secretions. Thus a truly hypoallergenic animal is, sadly, a myth. However, hope for some people may lie in hypoallergenic cat food, which dramatically reduces the amount of Fel d1 made by cats.[20] Time will tell whether this translates into a reduction in symptoms in cat-allergic humans, but it is a revolutionary and exciting concept.

Am I allergic to HDMs and/or pets?

If you are allergic to cats or dogs you will almost certainly know already: often just walking into a room where your four-legged friend has been sitting can be enough to set you off. As well as experiencing nasal symptoms, your eyes may itch and water.

HDM allergy is trickier and usually requires specific testing to diagnose it with certainty. The difference in response is because the particles that carry cat and dog allergen are small and therefore cause rapid symptoms, compared to the larger particles that carry HDM allergen. If after reading this chapter you think you **might be mite-allergic**, do get tested before undertaking avoidance measures; and do not become one of the many patients I have seen who have made huge efforts to reduce levels of HDM, only to discover they are not allergic at all. One of the saddest conversations I had was with a mother who had spent all her hard-earned savings on replacing carpets, bedding and curtains with laminate, a new mattress and dust-mite-proof covers and blinds, only to discover that her teenage son had non-allergic rhinitis and it wasn't dust-mite allergic at all.

4. Please Make It Stop: Treating Rhinitis and Hay Fever

Case study: my mother

When I was a child, my mother was extremely allergic to grass pollen. From May to July her eyes would itch and swell, her nose would run and our car windows were jammed shut to keep the pollen out while we all sweltered inside. My uncle would offer her his motorbike helmet so that she could go outside in spring and summer – she was not enamoured with this idea, and unsurprisingly she declined! Antihistamines made her sleepy, nose sprays didn't work and she did not want to bother her family doctor with something so 'minor'.

It was only when I began to train as an allergist that my mother finally got proper treatment and her symptoms vanished. It was a painful realization that so many summers had been unnecessarily spoilt. Since then I have met countless people who, like my mother, assume they should simply put up with their symptoms.

I want us to change things. Yes, 'us'. If you are reading this and recognize yourself from the story about my mother, or know someone with uncontrolled allergic rhinitis, I want you to know there is something that can be done. This chapter is all about treating allergic rhinitis: what works, what doesn't and the order in which you should try treatments.

Treatment steps

Allergists often break down the treatment of allergic rhinitis into five stages or 'steps' of treatment (see the illustration below). When a patient attends our clinic because treatment has not worked and their rhinitis is uncontrollable, we usually check that they have worked through these steps. Treatment is generally successful and, as you will see, there are many options.

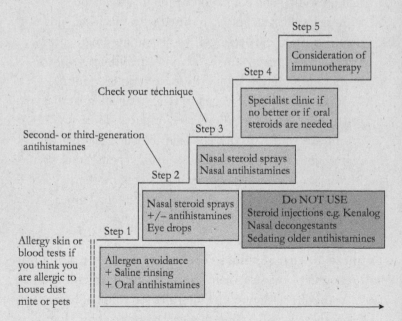

Treatment steps in allergic rhinitis

- **Step 1**: This involves a trio of allergen avoidance, nasal rinsing with saline and oral antihistamines. In my experience, antihistamines will almost always have been tried (for more on how to choose one to suit you, see page 54). Allergen avoidance will sometimes have been tried. However, awareness tends to be low when it comes to the benefits of saline rinsing. In pregnant women, who often prefer not to take any medication, saline rinses **alone** have been shown to reduce the symptoms of allergic rhinitis.[1]
- **Step 2**: This consists of an anti-inflammatory nasal steroid spray. The importance of this class of drugs cannot be overstated. If used correctly, they are highly effective in reducing **all** nasal symptoms and may also relieve itching, watery eyes. They work by reducing nasal inflammation. Some patients may also add in antihistamine eye drops if the intranasal steroid spray and antihistamine tablets are not enough.
- **Step 3**: If oral antihistamines and nasal corticosteroids do not provide good relief, then a combination nasal spray should be tried. These contain two drugs: an intranasal antihistamine and an intranasal steroid can be prescribed by your family doctor.
- **Step 4**: If you aren't getting any relief, your family doctor will probably refer you to an allergy specialist. However, most doctors will not generally refer you until some basic measures have been tried. The first thing that will happen in a clinic is that your specialist will check the previous three steps, to see if they have been followed correctly. So if you are invited to attend a clinic, do bring with you a list of all the medications you have tried.

- **Finally:** If all else fails, immunotherapy may be considered, if your allergy is severe and persistent.

In the rest of this chapter I will take you through the different steps in greater detail. I will also talk you through some 'red flag' drugs to avoid, plus other add-on treatments.

> <u>**Myth-buster: can honey cure my hay fever?**</u>
> **Sadly, there is no truth in the belief that the pollen present in honey desensitizes you, thus reducing the symptoms of hay fever. Honey is made by bees using the pollen from flowers, not from the pollen present in weeds, grasses and trees that typically trigger allergic-rhinitis symptoms.**

Allergen avoidance tactics

Avoid what you are allergic to – sounds simple, right? Sadly, avoidance isn't always straightforward with allergic rhinitis. Avoiding inhalant allergens completely can be tricky, but here are some simple strategies that can make a real difference.

If you have a pollen allergy

- **Stay inside** if possible, with the doors and windows closed, when the pollen count is highest. The pollen count is the amount of pollen per cubic metre observed during the previous twenty-four hours, which, when combined with weather conditions, provides the pollen forecast.[2]
- **Don't hang your washing outdoors** when the pollen count is high: pollen sticks to washing.

- **Shower before bed**: leave the pollen outside.
- **Sunglasses** significantly reduce symptoms in users with allergic rhinitis, and for some patients their impact is so significant that they need fewer antihistamine tablets.[3]
- **Keep car windows closed** when the pollen count is high, and use the car's air conditioning instead. Vacuum the interior regularly to remove pollen.
- **Consider low-pollen destinations** when booking your summer holiday, such as by the sea, where stronger ocean breezes can help blow allergens away.

Some of my patients tell me that air purifiers placed by their bed at night have reduced their symptoms, but there are no large convincing clinical trials to support their use.

If you have HDM allergy

While the following steps can reduce your exposure and symptoms, it is impossible to eradicate HDMs completely, leading a colleague to declare, 'I might as well go home, burn my mattress and sleep in a hammock!' Crucially, before understanding reduction measures it is important to have testing to confirm your allergy, as for measures to have any chance of working you need to get levels low enough to reduce symptoms. This can be time-consuming and expensive if you are investing in a new mattress and bedding. However, if you are going all out, here are some tips.

- **HDMs love warm, damp conditions**, so consider turning the heating down a few degrees, especially in your bedroom. Keep damp conditions to a minimum by using the extractor fan when having a bath or shower.

- **Use allergy-proof, removable covers** made from tightly woven material that make it harder for dust mites to invade your mattresses and pillow. While these will reduce levels of HDM allergen, studies show they do not lead to a reduction in symptoms, probably because one single measure is not enough.[4]

- **Put your bedding (mattress covers, sheets and blankets) on a weekly hot wash**: a 2008 study found that washing laundry at 60°C (140°F) kills all HDMs.[5]

- **Remove carpets if possible** (consider rugs or laminate) and avoid upholstered furniture.[6]

- **Dusting and vacuuming** disrupt the dust, allergens and debris, but using a damp cloth will absorb them better.

- **A high-efficiency particulate air (HEPA) filter** on your vacuum cleaner will trap the smallest particles.

- **A dehumidifier** helps to draw out some of the moisture that HDMs love.

Antihistamines

Antihistamines are drugs that block the effects of histamine and, in turn, relieve the symptoms caused by histamine release, such as nasal itching and itchy eyes. They also help to reduce a runny nose and sneezing, but are less effective at relieving nasal congestion.

Antihistamines are divided into types, known as generations. First-generation antihistamines are the oldest type; they cross into the brain and, as a result, can lead to drowsiness.

Their ability to help us sleep is why they often also make their way into over-the-counter cold and flu remedies. First-generation antihistamines include:

- **Chlorpheniramine** (found in the UK brand Piriton)
- **Diphenhydramine** (found in the US brand Benadryl – not to be confused with the UK brand of the same name*)
- **Promethazine** (found in Phenergan in Australia).

Second- and third-generation antihistamines are the newer successors, with one key difference: they don't cross into the brain as easily (if at all) and so are far less likely to cause drowsiness.

Don't be DIM: why first-generation antihistamines are best avoided

First-generation antihistamines are classed as driving-impairment medication (DIM). Not only do they cross the blood–brain barrier, sedating us, but studies also show that they are less effective than the newer second- or third-generation antihistamines.[7]

In 2000 University of Iowa doctors looked at the impact of first-generation antihistamines on driving performance, using a driving simulator.[8] They discovered that the group who took the first-generation antihistamines were more impaired when driving than the group who were legally drunk. Worryingly,

---

* Benadryl sold in the UK contains the second-generation antihistamines – acrivastine for adults (Benadryl Relief) and cetirizine for children (Benadryl Allergy Children).

the group taking diphenhydramine did not always feel sleepy, thereby calling into question whether drivers can safely judge if they are fit to drive after taking it.

It is not only drowsiness and potential driving impairment that are concerning. Children are still frequently prescribed syrups containing first-generation antihistamines and can become hyper (instead of drowsy) after taking them. And in the elderly their use can trigger delirium. One study has even linked long-term first-generation antihistamine use to an increased chance of developing dementia and Alzheimer's disease.[9]

Rhinitis guidelines for healthcare professionals universally state that first-generation antihistamines should be avoided, and yet these drugs remain widely sold and used across the world.

> **Go for ingredients, not brand name**
> **When buying an antihistamine, look at the name of the active drug, not the brand name. Sometimes the antihistamine will be marketed under several different brand names, but as long as the drug is the same, you won't go wrong.**

Choosing the right antihistamine for you

There is a huge array of over-the-counter and prescription antihistamines. It is down to personal choice, but I recommend trying a second- or third-generation antihistamine because they are longer-acting and are usually non-sedating (although there is individual variation in how susceptible you are to drowsiness).

Acrivastine, loratadine, cetirizine, fexofenadine, desloratadine, levocetirizine and bilastine are the most common second- and third-generation antihistamines. Acrivastine is the fastest-acting, but needs to be taken every eight hours and therefore few allergy specialists recommend it. Fexofenadine is the least likely to cause drowsiness and is a popular choice. It is available to buy over the counter in the USA, Australia and New Zealand, and in certain European countries, including the UK since October 2021. In addition, according to the US Food and Drug Administration (FDA), grapefruit, apple and orange juice may all interfere with its action, so if you do use it, do not take it with fruit juice. I usually recommend cetirizine to my patients as it is highly effective, has a fast onset of action, a long duration and is widely available.

What about children? Dr Paul Turner, a world-famous researcher and reader in paediatric allergy and immunology at Imperial College London says, 'Although cetirizine is licensed for children over two years, in practice cetirizine is used in children over one year of age as there is very good safety data.[10] It is often used in younger children too, but only on medical advice. So if you have a very young child who needs antihistamines, you should discuss with your doctor which antihistamine they would recommend.'

Saline rinsing

Also known as nasal irrigation or nasal douching, a saline rinse involves rinsing your nasal passages with a salt-water solution, using an aerosolized spray, a saline rinse bottle or a device called a netipot. It seems strange that rinsing your nose out with a saline mist, or a fat, squeezy bottle or teapot-like contraption, will reduce the symptoms of allergic rhinitis, but somehow it does. It is thought that it thins the mucus in the nose and removes allergens lodged in your nostril.

I believe that saline rinses both help to clear the mucus and allow steroid nasal sprays to be better absorbed as a result, and for this reason I recommend them to patients. There are various preparations that can be bought over the counter or online; in some cases the spray is already made up, and in others you add cool boiled water to a pre-prepared sachet of sodium chloride and sodium bicarbonate.

Nasal steroid sprays

Nasal steroid sprays are highly effective at reducing all nasal symptoms of allergic rhinitis, such as sneezing, a runny nose, itchy eyes and nasal congestion. This is because they reduce the influx of inflammatory cells into the lining of the nose when you are exposed to an allergen and block the release of inflammatory chemicals. Unlike antihistamines, which try to limit the damage from allergens after exposure has occurred, nasal steroid sprays are a preventative treatment. Think of these drugs as the 'police force' in allergic rhinitis – stopping the party from even getting started, or breaking it up if in full swing. Some can be bought over the counter, while others are prescription-only.

Don't be put off by the word 'steroid': newer nasal sprays containing the steroids mometasone furoate (Nasonex), fluticasone furoate (Avamys) and fluticasone propionate

(Flixonase) are barely absorbed into the circulation, meaning that side-effects such as thinning of the bones are minimal.

Other nasal steroids, such as beclomethasone, budesonide and triamcinolone, do have a higher absorption rate, but are safe for long-term use. A specialist may prescribe a short course of a spray or drops containing betamethasone, but it should not be used long-term.

Why technique matters: mastering the art of using a nasal steroid spray

Patients often tell me that they have tried nasal steroid sprays without success. When we explore this, it is generally because they have been using it incorrectly or have stopped too soon. So let me share with you a few tricks of the trade (see the illustration overleaf).

Nasal steroid sprays take a while to build up: some people may find relief within a day or two, but it often takes up to two weeks to notice a difference. If you have hay fever, start using the spray about two weeks before the start of the hay-fever season. If you begin to use them before your nose becomes stuffy and runny, they will nip any allergic inflammation in the bud and work much better. If your child struggles with a nasal spray, try gently using it when he or she is asleep.

The most common side-effect of sprays is nosebleeds. If this happens, take a break for a few days and then try again. When using the spray, always ensure it is angled towards the side wall of the nose and not the septum (the partition between the nostrils). If the bleeding recurs, pop

1. Wash your nose out with a saline rinse. Wait two to three minutes.

2. Looking down, take the spray in your **right** hand and place the nozzle just inside your **left** nostril, taking care not to direct the nozzle towards the septum. This means the spray will land on the side wall of the nose, improving its effectiveness and also reducing the likelihood of a nosebleed.

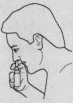

3. Aiming the spray towards the outside wall, squirt the spray into your nostril. Then take the spray in your **left** hand and repeat with your **right** nostril.

4. Don't sniff after squirting the spray. This is one of the biggest reasons for treatment failure. Instead, just breathe in and out gently. One tip is to brush your teeth immediately after using the nose spray, as this will often reduce the urge to sniff.

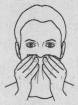

5. If the spray drips out, dab with a tissue, but again do not sniff.

How to use a nasal spray correctly

a blob of Vaseline, using your little fingertip, on the septum just inside the nostril. Moisturization can help to reduce the bleeding. You may find that Avamys works best if you are prone to nosebleeds, because of the shorter nozzle and finer spray.

In my experience, 90 per cent of patients will find that their symptoms of allergic rhinitis improve significantly if they follow the advice I have described. If symptoms persist, then other treatments (see below) may be needed and it is time to consider specialist help.

Dymista

Dymista is a combination nasal spray containing a steroid called fluticasone propionate and a very fast-acting antihistamine called azelastine. The antihistamine reduces itching, sneezing, a runny nose and eye symptoms, while the steroid acts on the cells in the nasal lining and reduces their production of inflammatory chemicals. Interestingly the combination works better than the two drugs used separately and helps both the nasal symptoms and itchy, sore eyes.[11] Dymista is prescription-only in the UK and is not recommended for children under twelve.

Anti-leukotrienes: montelukast and zafirlukast

These are prescription-only medicines normally used as an add-on treatment in asthma, but in adults and children with asthma who also have troublesome rhinitis, specialists will often give them a trial. They work by blocking highly inflammatory chemicals called leukotrienes, which are released by the body in response to allergens, causing inflammation in the nose and airways.

Drugs to avoid

- **Nasal decongestants**: You would think nasal decongestants would be useful in treating a stuffy allergic nose, but the opposite can be true. They do nothing to get rid of the allergic inflammation that is causing the nasal blockage and, when used for more than a few days, can cause a rebound swelling in the nose known as rhinitis medicamentosa. I have seen many patients caught in a vicious cycle of feeling blocked due to allergy, using a decongestant and initially feeling better, but then developing rebound blockage that is worse than ever. So they reach for the decongestants and the cycle continues. The main culprits are decongestants such as xylometazoline and oxymetazoline found in cold and flu remedies.

  My advice is never to use nasal decongestant sprays for more than seventy-two hours, even though they may be marketed alongside anthistamines to treat allergic rhinitis. If you are currently using them, don't worry. Talk to your doctor about stopping gradually. Your doctor may suggest introducing a nasal steroid spray at the same time, or even a short course of oral steroids if your congestion is very bad, to take the edge off things while you are reducing their use.

- **Depot (slow-release) steroid injections**: Another group of drugs to avoid are depot steroid injections such as triamcinolone (trade name Kenalog). These are usually injected into the buttock and the drug is slowly released into the bloodstream.

Triamcinolone is incredibly effective at relieving hay-fever symptoms and used to be commonly prescribed, but it has fallen out of fashion due to a concerning side-effect profile including diabetes, muscle weakness, changes in mood, weight gain and osteoporosis or thinning of the bones. I have seen the devastating consequences of these side-effects, including in a forty-eight-year-old taxi driver who fractured his wrist and consequently lost his job, after developing osteoporosis from years of regular triamcinolone injections. UK rhinitis guidelines do not recommend their use. Oral steroids are a potential option, but there are far better long-term options available, such as allergen immunotherapy (see below).

If it is getting to the point where you are thinking about asking for these injections, then your family doctor should be referring you to see an allergist.

Allergen immunotherapy (AIT)

For a minority of patients, all of the previous steps will not be enough to manage symptoms, and AIT – also known as allergen desensitization – may be needed. It is offered to patients in whom rhinitis due to pollens (such as grass, birch and ragweed), HDM and animals such as cats and dogs cannot be controlled by medication.

Case study: Adam

In the early 1900s two young doctors, Leonard Noon and John Freeman, were working hard in their laboratories at St Mary's Hospital (where I now work) on a pioneering new treatment. They were injecting an extract of grass pollen under the skin to treat patients with hay fever. The treatment worked, and in 1911 they published their work in *The Lancet* medical journal. They are both credited as the inventors of allergen desensitization. Sadly, Noon died two years later from pulmonary tuberculosis, leaving Freeman to continue their work alone. By 1954 my mentor, William Frankland, was working for Freeman and performed the first *de rigueur* trial of grass-pollen immunotherapy that year, establishing a firm scientific foundation for this treatment.

Fast-forward to 2020, and my ten-year-old nephew Adam has terrible hay fever, and standard medical treatments are not touching it. So I suggest that his parents ask their family doctor for a referral to see my colleagues in paediatric allergy at St Mary's. Most people with rhinitis will find that antihistamines and/or an intranasal steroid spray will sort them out: for example, Adam's younger sister Sara also has hay fever and is fine with tablets.

However, some patients like Adam will not respond and so are referred to an allergy clinic. In this group we will usually 'optimize' their treatment, but if they still continue to suffer, then we can try and help with AIT, as my colleagues did with Adam.

So how does AIT work? Surely giving someone an extract of what they are allergic to would make things worse? Let's use grass pollen as an example. AIT to grass involves giving a potent extract of grass pollen in 'industrial' doses – about 2,000 times more than you would be exposed to during a pollen season – either by an injection into the arm or a daily tablet under the tongue over a period of three years. This reprograms the immune system by reducing the number of over-enthusiastic T-cells that are 'turned on' by grass pollen, and by encouraging B-cells to treat specific IgE to grass as the 'enemy' and produce blocking IgG (immunoglobulin G) antibodies that 'neutralize' it.[12]

The great thing is that as well as treating symptoms, AIT is a way of achieving long-term remission in rhinitis: in other words, it enables us to modify the natural history of the disease. So a three-year course of treatment usually enables patients to remain well for many years afterwards.[13]

The main risk of AIT is that the injections can very rarely cause a severe allergic reaction. Usually injections build up in strength and are either given over the course of the three years or more intensely clustered together before three consecutive pollen seasons. As a result of the risk of anaphylaxis, the treatment is given in hospital clinics and a wait of thirty to sixty minutes after each injection is recommended.

Tablet immunotherapy usually has only minor side-effects, such as an itchy mouth or slight swelling, but it does involve three years of daily treatment and is costly, which may limit its access for some individuals.

As for Adam, the addition of AIT to his usual medication means that his symptoms have melted away. He can now go and play football in the park with his friends and this summer went camping and had no hay-fever symptoms. His parents are relieved that his hay fever will not disrupt his studies. His life has transformed. I like to think the pioneers of allergen desensitization (Drs Noon, Freeman and Frankland), who all worked at St Mary's, would be smiling if they knew.

5. COVID-19 and Allergy

When I began writing this book back in 2020 I did not antici-pate including a chapter on COVID-19 and allergy. Like everyone else, I hoped the pandemic would be over within twelve months and that normal life would return. Sadly, it appears that SARS-CoV-2, and by extension COVID-19, are with us for the foreseeable future.

During the first wave, many allergists were redeployed to different areas while balancing continuing care for their allergy patients. Day-clinics physically closed their doors, but an army of allergists – me included – turned on their laptops and switched to remote consultations.

When the first UK COVID-19 vaccination was given on 8 December 2020 the nation breathed a collective sigh of relief. But then there were reports of allergic reactions to the vaccines, and so the speciality was thrust into the limelight. Within twenty-four hours the BSACI set up a COVID-19 vaccine-allergy group and I was invited to join. Those early days were both exciting and stressful. Fortunately, initial concerns that anaphylaxis could turn out to be a significant problem were not borne out, and severe allergic reactions have been extremely rare.

Vaccines are more than 95 per cent effective in reducing serious COVID-19 infection, including the Delta variant.[1,2] And they don't only protect us; they protect those around us and offer the most hope of restoring the normal life that we yearn for.

Many allergists, including me, rapidly set up COVID-19 vaccine-allergy clinics. Allergy teams across the world have been busier than ever. I found myself doing everything from offering guidance to colleagues, to writing Frequently Asked Questions for family doctors and reviewing statements about the COVID-19 vaccine and anaphylaxis from the World Allergy Organization Anaphylaxis Committee. It has been hugely satisfying to know that I have made a meaningful contribution to the fight against COVID-19.

In this chapter I will answer the most common questions that I have been asked about allergy and COVID-19, and I will offer some practical tips and coping strategies.

Does having an allergy put me more at risk of COVID-19?

No. Having an allergy neither increases the likelihood of catching COVID-19 nor puts you at risk of developing more severe symptoms if you do.

Initially there were concerns that asthmatics would be more poorly than non-asthmatics, because respiratory viral infections often trigger asthma. However, it transpired that, unlike most respiratory viruses, COVID-19 appears to have a limited effect on the airways of asthmatics. Patients with asthma are not more vulnerable to catching COVID-19, nor are they more likely to be hospitalized.[3] Children with asthma are also not at increased risk of severe COVID-19 infection.

I have rhinitis and asthma. Are steroid nasal sprays and inhaled corticosteroids (ICS) still safe to use, should I catch COVID-19?

Stopping steroid nasal sprays for rhinitis is not recommended. As well as your rhinitis becoming worse if you stop them, uncontrolled sneezing is a great way to spread infection. Furthermore, using steroid nasal sprays has been found to be associated with a lower risk of COVID-19-related hospitalization, intensive-care admission and death. Further studies are now planned.[4] It is less clear if ICS in asthmatics may also have a protective effect against COVID-19; surprisingly, early data suggests that asthmatics admitted to hospital with COVID-19 are likely to do better than non-asthmatic patients, but more studies are expected.[5]

The best way of reducing the potential severity of COVID-19, if you have asthma, is by ensuring that your asthma is as well controlled as possible. Check that your asthma treatment plan is up-to-date and that you are taking your inhalers regularly, as prescribed. If you have an exacerbation of asthma and are prescribed a short course of oral steroids, then you should take them, regardless of whether you are COVID-19 positive or not.

Is it hay fever – or COVID-19?

Navigating the pollen season during COVID-19 is tricky, and of course people with allergies can also catch COVID-19. As you can see from the diagram overleaf, many symptoms of hay fever and COVID-19 overlap. The only definitive way to answer this question is by taking a COVID-19 test.

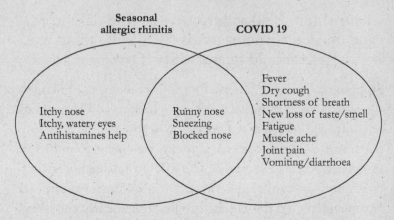

Symptoms of seasonal allergic rhinitis and COVID-19

It is worth bearing in mind that if it is hay fever, then anti-allergy medications should bring relief. In addition, mask-wearing has been scientifically proven to reduce the symptoms of hay fever.[6] In contrast, symptoms of COVID-19 will not respond to antihistamines or nasal sprays and you are more likely to feel generally unwell.

Some people with hay fever are concerned that their symptoms will be mistaken for COVID-19 when out in public. My advice? This time is as good as any to get your symptoms of hay fever as well controlled as possible.

COVID-19 vaccines and allergy

Data suggests that 999,992 people out of a million will receive their vaccination without developing a severe allergic reaction.[7] At the time of writing, an incredible 7 billion vaccine doses have been administered globally (the world population is a little under eight billion) and there are no reports of fatal anaphylactic reactions to the COVID-19 vaccine. Those who have reacted have made a full recovery.

However, even though allergic reactions to the vaccines are vanishingly rare, the initial publicity generated when allergic reactions to the Pfizer BioNTech vaccine in the UK were reported understandably led to concern among people with allergies. The rare episodes of blood clots and unusual bleeding after the AstraZeneca COVID-19 vaccine, especially in younger people, were not due to an allergic reaction to the vaccine or driven by an allergic mechanism. Here I want to reassure and answer some of the FAQs that I get asked about COVID-19 vaccines and allergy.

However, these FAQs are **not** a substitute for a discussion with your family doctor if you have concerns about allergy and your individual health.

Are people with allergies at increased risk of developing an allergy to the COVID-19 vaccines?

There is no evidence that people with allergic conditions such as asthma, hay fever, food or insect-sting allergy are at greater risk of vaccine allergy compared to the general population.

What about drug allergies specifically?

If you have had an anaphylactic reaction to a medicine – including antibiotics, anaesthetics and painkillers – and the trigger has been identified, you can receive the vaccination.

Previous reactions to vaccines are slightly more complicated, and if you have had anaphylaxis to a vaccine, then your family doctor should liaise with an allergy clinic. However, historically no vaccines have contained the additive polyethylene glycol (PEG) and only a few have contained polysorbate 80 (see below). So even if you have previously developed a severe allergic reaction to a vaccine, you should be able to be vaccinated against COVID-19, although you may be advised to have that first vaccine in a hospital setting. If you have had a severe allergic reaction to the first dose of a COVID-19 vaccine or you have a known allergy to PEG or polysorbate 80, then a referral to a specialist is advised.

What are PEG and polysorbate 80?

PEGs are a group of additives (the medical term for this is 'excipient') commonly found in medicines, including antihistamines, antibiotics and painkillers, plus many household products and cosmetics. They are also called macrogols. The Pfizer BioNTech and Moderna mRNA vaccines contain polyethylene glycol 2000 (PEG).

Polysorbate 80 (also known as Tween 80) is also widely added to medicines, including some flu vaccines. It is a stabilizer or emulsifier. It can be added to foods, such as ice-creams and other dairy-based puddings, to keep their creamy texture without them separating. The AstraZeneca, Janssen and Sputnik vaccines all contain polysorbate 80.

Allergy to either excipient is exceptionally rare.

Why do some people develop allergic reactions?

Truthfully, we don't know. Usually when someone is allergic to a medicine or food they will react whenever they take it, but we are finding that people who had an allergic reaction to the first dose of the COVID-19 vaccine can almost always tolerate the second,[8] even if that reaction was fairly severe. There were initial concerns that people who reacted might be allergic to PEG or polysorbate 80. However, allergy testing has so far shown that an allergy to the excipients has been very much the exception and not the rule.

How do I know if I am allergic to PEG or polysorbate 80?

If you are allergic to either additive, then it is likely that you already know. Usually PEG-allergic patients have a history of severe anaphylaxis, requiring hospital admission within two hours of receiving unrelated drugs, such as long-acting steroid injections or laxatives that contain high molecular-weight PEGs. If you are unsure whether or not you may be allergic, do ask your family doctor for advice.

I had an anaphylactic reaction, but the cause wasn't found – can I be vaccinated?

Anaphylaxis without an identifiable trigger is not usually a reason to avoid the vaccine, but your family doctor will probably check with a specialist.

I developed a large red area of swelling at the site of my COVID-19 vaccination? Does that mean I am allergic?

Mild pain and tenderness are common side-effects of the vaccine. Delayed swelling and redness developing four to eleven days after the vaccine and lasting for more than a week are also normal, especially with the Moderna vaccine. If this happens to you, take an antihistamine for the itching, such as cetirizine. You can use paracetamol and ice-packs to relieve discomfort. You can still receive a second dose in the community but, to be ultra-safe, UK guidance advises that you should be observed for thirty minutes after vaccination. Allergy testing is not needed.

I have a latex allergy. Will the vaccine syringe contain latex?

The manufacturers of the Pfizer BioNTech, AstraZeneca, Moderna and Janssen COVID-19 vaccines all advise that the injection vial does not contain latex.

6. An Introduction to Food Allergies

When you or someone close to you has a food allergy, the simple act of sustenance can become a veritable mine-field. Open the cupboards in any kitchen and you'll be greeted by an array of tins, packets and pouches listing dozens of ingredients with often unfamiliar and bewildering names. This can make adhering to the first line of defence against food allergy – avoidance of the culprit food – a real challenge.

Yet according to the European Academy of Allergy and Clinical Immunology (EAACI), for every person who has a food allergy, there will be another six people who believe that they are allergic.[1] One study assessed 969 young children for food allergy and, while 34.7 per cent of parents reported a food-related problem, only around 5 per cent of the children were actually allergic.[2]

This overestimate occurs for two main reasons. Access to allergy clinics is often limited, making it difficult to reach a diagnosis, and allergy tests do not give a clear-cut 'yes or no' answer as to whether you are allergic or not. I have seen many patients who have been mistakenly diagnosed with a food allergy based on a blood test. Furthermore, we live in a world where increasingly we are very quick to point the finger at food. Scarcely a day passes without one ingredient or another being extolled as a superfood, or vilified as the cause of allergy or intolerance. Supermarkets have been quick to cash in on this trend, with a huge expansion in 'free from' ranges.

The good news is that if you are struggling to identify which food is driving your symptoms, then you probably do not have a food allergy. If you have a food allergy, you will usually know the culprit food and react every time you eat enough of it (for the rare exceptions to this rule, see Chapter 8).

Doctors will classify reactions to foods into toxic and non-toxic. Most of us will have suffered the misfortune of a 'toxic' reaction, like food poisoning, at some point. Certain types of food poisoning can even mimic food allergy – the best known is scombroid (see below).

Scombroid food poisoning

The scombridae comprise a family of fish that we eat frequently and are well known. They include mackerel, tuna, mahi-mahi, marlin and bonito. If, when they are caught, they are not refrigerated properly, an overgrowth of bacteria can lead to high levels of histamine building up in the flesh of the fish. So if a person eats the fish, they may develop symptoms that are identical to an allergic reaction. Symptoms can begin as quickly as five minutes after eating or may be delayed for up to two hours. Often the fish has a metallic taste at the time of eating it. Symptoms usually last up to twenty-four hours, and in severe cases people may need to attend A&E for anti-sickness medication and fluids.

The remainder of food reactions are non-toxic and may be:

- Immune and due to the presence of specific IgE to a food – namely, a food allergy
- Immune and not due to the presence of specific IgE to a food (see Chapter 8)
- Not driven by our immune system – namely, a food intolerance (see Chapter 1).

Time for food allergy 101

Food allergy is a huge and important area, and patients will often come to my clinic armed with a list of questions – and these may be questions that you want answers to as well.

How common is food allergy?

The World Allergy Organization estimates that food allergy affects 2.5 per cent of people globally. Figures range from 1 to 10 per cent, depending on the country, as testing for food allergy is complicated and access to specialist clinics to confirm a diagnosis varies between countries. However, data suggest that levels of food allergy are significantly lower in China (including Hong Kong), Russia and India compared to Europe, the US and Australasia.[3]

Which foods most commonly cause food allergy?

The most common food allergies in children are due to eggs, cow's milk and peanuts, while fresh fruits, peanuts, tree nuts and shellfish dominate in adults.[4] Around 90 per cent of anaphylactic reactions are to proteins in the following foods:

- Peanut
- Tree nuts
- Cow's milk protein (CMP)
- Hen's egg
- Fish
- Prawns
- Soya
- Wheat
- Sesame.

However, pretty much any food protein can cause an allergic reaction (I have treated patients with anaphylaxis to foods as diverse as bee pollen, asparagus and fish roe). Fats or carbohydrates do not cause allergic reactions, with the lone exception of the sugar galactose-alpha-1,3-galactose (alpha-gal),which causes red-meat allergy (see Chapter 7).

In addition, true IgE-mediated allergy to food additives like E-numbers is exceptionally rare, and cases are self-reported rather than proven. The one exception is the red food colouring carmine (used in red-velvet cupcakes, yoghurts and soft drinks), which is actually made from crushing an insect called cochineal. The protein-rich colouring is a known cause of anaphylaxis.[5]

The good news is that the levels of food allergy in many parts of the world may be starting to stabilize: a 2018 Australian study found that prevalence of food sensitization had not significantly changed in infants over fifteen years; and while sensitization is not the same as allergy, it would be surprising if levels of sensitization stayed the same while allergy increased.[6] Meanwhile in the UK, despite the increase in food anaphylaxis, the fatality rate has plummeted by almost 80 per cent.[7] So if you suffer a reaction you are more likely than ever before to survive.

However, as nobody can predict who will die from an anaphylactic reaction to food, and food is a daily part of our lives, a diagnosis of food allergy often fuels stress, anxiety and social isolation. Day-to-day activities, such as shopping and cooking, can take far longer and have an added layer of complication. Every few months a heart-breaking case of someone dying from a food allergy (usually a child or teenager) will make its way into the headlines, not only increasing awareness of the potential seriousness of the condition, but

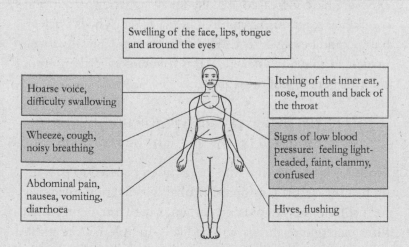

Any combination of these symptoms may occur. The shaded boxes are the signs that tip a reaction over into anaphylaxis.

What are the symptoms of food allergy?

also – as I am all too aware – increasing fear among patients and their families.

Which foods are most likely to cause severe allergic reactions?

On one level, if you have a food allergy, the answer to this question does not really matter. What matters is having the tools and strategies to reduce the risk of a reaction from your own trigger food. However, peanuts, walnuts and hazelnuts are the common cause of fatal reactions in adults and children in the UK and Europe. Yet it is cow's milk protein (CMP) that is the biggest cause for concern among allergists like myself. Over the last twenty years deaths due to accidental CMP exposure have increased, making up a staggering 26 per cent of all fatal reactions in children in the UK.[8] Why is unclear, but it could be down to CMP being present, and often well hidden, in so many foods. CMP is found in everything from chewing gum to hot dogs.

Is it true that every allergic reaction I have to a food will be worse than the last one?

No! This is a myth, and one that is often peddled to patients by healthcare professionals, probably reflecting a lack of formal training. There is no certain way of predicting what future allergic reactions will be like. Multiple factors influence the severity of an allergic reaction, including the amount of food consumed, whether you have asthma, and the speed at which you receive adrenaline. Your 'threshold dose' will also influence the severity of a reaction. Let me explain more: imagine that you are a high-jumper and are about to jump over the bar. Think of that bar as the amount of allergen that you would need to eat, in order to develop an allergic reaction. This is your 'threshold dose' and it varies from person to person. For example, the average peanut contains 300mg of potentially allergy-inducing peanut protein. Some people may react if they eat 30mg, while for others it could just take 3mg to trigger a reaction. Studies have shown that tiredness and exercise can dramatically lower your threshold dose,[9] so you react to far less allergen; and we suspect that viral illness, NSAIDs (non-steroidal anti-inflammatory drugs), alcohol and stress also reduce your threshold dose.

Can I be 'screened' for food allergies?

World-famous paediatric allergist Professor David Stukus, of the Nationwide Children's Hospital in Ohio, wrote on Twitter, 'I spend considerable time undiagnosing food allergy incorrectly diagnosed by inappropriate testing. I feel so bad for these families thinking that they are allergic when they are not.'

This a scenario that every allergist can relate to. The first and the most important part of diagnosing a food allergy is a detailed and comprehensive medical history. This is the reference point against which subsequent skin-prick tests and specific IgE blood tests are interpreted. Although these tests are essential in confirming a diagnosis of food allergy, it requires skill to interpret them; and unlike a pregnancy test, they don't give a clear-cut positive/negative result. False positives are common, particularly in patients with eczema, who have high levels of total IgE, which interferes with allergy blood tests. False negatives are also not unheard of. The size of a skin-prick test or the levels of specific IgE will also not predict the severity of an allergic reaction, but will give a reasonable idea of the likelihood of allergy.

So if someone offers you 'allergy screening', hastily beat a retreat. Indiscriminate testing is possibly the worst thing you can do. I have had patients who have needlessly cut out entire food groups as a result of inappropriate testing, when they aren't actually allergic.

Should I get tested for food intolerances and sensitivities?

Searching for 'food-intolerance testing' online throws up thousands of sites and clinics offering their services, but please don't waste your money. Tests including Vega testing (electrodiagnostic), kinesiology, bioresonance to foods and IgG testing are expensive and unproven.

> **Why you should give IgG blood tests a wide berth**
> One of the most widely available tests online with no scientific backing is IgG testing. Companies offer the enticing prospect of being tested for more than 200 foods that you might encounter. It is comprehensive, but also meaningless; blood is tested for IgG antibodies rather than IgE antibodies, which are the cause of food allergies. The presence of IgG signifies exposure to a food, not an allergy,

and indicates what you have been eating recently and not whether it is doing any harm. A positive IgG test to a food is a sign of a normal immune system, and a positive result may actually indicate tolerance for the food, not intolerance. If you think you have an undiagnosed food allergy, speak to your family doctor, who can refer you to an allergy clinic if appropriate (see Chapter 13).

Will my child outgrow their food allergy?

Most children will outgrow allergies to milk, egg, wheat and soya by the time they reach school age, whereas only 10–20 per cent will outgrow a nut allergy. For more about individual food allergens, see Appendix 1 (page 191).[10]

Can food allergy be cured?

Currently there is no 'cure' for food allergy, but there are treatments such as immunotherapy or desensitization to food, which can convince your immune system that a particular food is not a threat. The idea of this sort of treatment is to protect patients from developing anaphylaxis if they accidentally consume the food they are allergic to. So if someone with peanut allergy undergoes desensitization with peanut, they do not need to worry nearly as much about cross-contamination or eating out.

So how does it work? As with all immunotherapy, there are two stages: an initial up-dosing phase and a maintenance phase. During the up-dosing phase patients will gradually start to eat their allergenic food, such as peanut. They start with a minute dose and slowly increase it. This can be done over days in a hospital setting or over several weeks, where the initial doses are given in hospital and the later doses at home. Once the top dose is achieved, patients move on to the maintenance phase, where they continue taking the top dose for the rest of their life. In the case of peanut, this is around 300mg – or the amount of peanut protein in one kernel.

This regular exposure is required so that their immune system remains convinced that the food is not a threat. It is also not a treatment with a clear end, and to remain tolerant it may be that you will have to consume nuts, egg or milk (or whatever food you are being desensitized to) indefinitely – in contrast to venom immunotherapy, where at the end of a course of treatment most patients can consider themselves cured.

Deciding to attempt food-allergy desensitization is very much an individual decision. Some patients and their families absolutely love it, while others prefer to opt for avoidance (for pros and cons, see the table on page 83). Historically, in the UK, where there are so few trained allergists, desensitization has been largely confined to research settings but in 2020 both the US FDA and the European Commission approved Palforzia. This is a pharmaceutical-grade oral peanut immunotherapy tablet, which makes peanut desensitization easier for both patients and their allergists. There was further good news in December 2021, when NHS England agreed to offer Palforzia to up to 2,000 children. My hope is that it will translate into improved access within the NHS to peanut desensitization for those patients who are interested.

Pros and cons of food-allergy desensitization

Pros	Cons
A huge improvement in quality of life and reduction in anxiety levels. You can be more relaxed when eating or walking into environments where food is aerosolized, such as a coffee shop if you are allergic to CMP.	Anaphylaxis is more likely than if avoiding the food. This can be disconcerting, if you have managed for years without anaphylaxis. And if you have multiple reactions, it can negatively impact your quality of life.
Decreased risk of a severe life-threatening reaction from accidental exposure.	Chronic symptoms, such as abdominal pain, and mild reactions are more likely, which is unsurprising as you are consuming an allergenic food most days.
It is easier to introduce new foods into the diet, especially if avoiding 'may contains'.	As children get older, and especially as they hit their teen years, they do not want to stick to the schedule.
	It can be expensive and difficult to access.

7. Stranger than Fiction: Food Allergies You May Not Have Heard Of

We've covered the telltale signs of food allergy where a person accidentally eats a known allergen and suffers a reaction of varying degrees of severity. But some types of food allergy can be much more nuanced, or it may take a very specific set of circumstances to trigger a reaction.

From food allergies linked to hay fever, latex allergy and tick bites, to a patient of mine who was convinced she was allergic to New Year's Eve, in this chapter I will take you further into the fascinating world of food allergies.

Case study: Milo

Milo was a sixteen-year-old boy referred to me by his family doctor. Eating raw fruit made his mouth itch and his throat feel uncomfortable. Helping his parents prep the vegetables for Sunday lunch was out of the question, because peeling carrots, parsnips and potatoes made his hands itchy. Confusingly, Milo was able to eat apple pie and tinned peaches without any sign of a reaction, plus plenty of roasted carrots, potatoes and parsnips. Everyone was baffled, but in fact what Milo had was a classic case of pollen food syndrome (PFS), which affects about 2 per cent of people in the UK.[1]

Pollen food syndrome

PFS is a reaction to the proteins found in raw fruits, vegetables, some tree nuts and soya, which contain proteins similar in structure to proteins found in certain pollens (such as birch, mugwort, ragweed and grass). So when some people who are allergic to one of these pollens eats related foods, their immune system gets confused and thinks they are eating a mouthful of pollen. Reactions are usually mild, being limited to an itchy mouth, lips or ears, a slightly tight, itchy, uncomfortable throat or sneezing. Severe allergic reactions are rarer, and at least 90 per cent of patients will not need to carry adrenaline.

Cooking or canning the fruit, nut or vegetable will usually destroy the cross-reactive protein – which explains why Milo could eat baked apple pie to his heart's content, but would react after eating fresh apples.

Birch pollen is the most common cause of PFS in the UK and Europe. About two-thirds of birch-pollen-allergic people will develop PFS, usually to seeded or stoned fruit and less often to soya or root vegetables. In the US and Canada, where allergy to ragweed pollen is common, cross-reactivity between ragweed and foods such as banana, cucumber, melon, sunflower seeds and courgettes is also a problem. In Eastern Europe, PFS is seen more frequently in people who are allergic to mugwort pollen (which can cross-react to proteins found in celery, carrots and some spices). Rarely PFS is also triggered by grass pollen (which can cross-react with raw tomato, melon or peaches).

How is PFS diagnosed?

It's important to distinguish between pollen-related and non-pollen-related food allergy. If you suspect you might have PFS, you need to see an allergist, who will take a detailed history and then can confirm the diagnosis using skin testing and blood tests. Your allergist will look at your history test results and the severity of previous reactions, when deciding whether or not you need injectable adrenaline. Patients with PFS will not react to every single raw fruit, vegetable or nut that shares similar proteins to pollen, so should only avoid a food if it provokes a reaction.

If soya is your trigger or if you are unsure whether you are allergic, avoid soya milk, soya yoghurts and puddings that contain large amounts of soya protein.

> **<u>Navigating PFS</u>**
> **If you have PFS, avoid freshly made fruit smoothies or freshly squeezed juices made from the fruits or vegetables or nuts you are allergic to. That is because drinking rather than eating the offending fruit or vegetable can trigger a more severe reaction, as you are rapidly exposed to a large amount of concentrated allergen. Smoothies and fruit juices in supermarket chiller sections are usually fine as they are pasteurized. Take particular care with foods during the pollen season because, in many patients, symptoms worsen during the season of the pollen in question. One way to eliminate symptoms is to bake or microwave the food, because high temperatures**

will destroy the proteins responsible for PFS. Eating canned food may also limit the reaction. And peeling the fruit or vegetable before eating may be helpful, as the offending protein is often concentrated in the skin.

<u>Latex-fruit syndrome</u>

Latex is a natural rubber collected from the sap of the rubber tree, which can cause allergic reactions. Levels of latex allergy have fallen dramatically in the last twenty years, as we use it less frequently today. Nowadays the main exposure people have to latex comes from condoms and balloons, or from medical equipment such as sterile gloves and some urinary catheters.

An estimated 30–50 per cent of people with latex allergy are affected by latex-fruit syndrome.[2] Like PFS and pollen, the proteins found in some fruits are similar to latex, triggering allergic symptoms. Common cross-reactive fruits include avocado, banana, kiwi fruit, passion fruit and chestnuts. Reactions can vary in severity and, as with PFS, cross-reactive fruits do not have to be routinely avoided unless they cause problems.

Food-dependent exercise-induced anaphylaxis (FDEIA)

Exercise is essential for healthy living, but for some patients that I see, it could be fatal under certain conditions. FDEIA was first described in 1979 in a long-distance runner living in Denver,

Colorado, who suffered allergic reactions of varying severity.[3] His allergist made the connection that it was the combination of eating shellfish and going on a run several hours later that was the problem. So the man stopped eating shellfish before running and never suffered from anaphylaxis again.

The cause of FDEIA is not entirely clear, but the dominant theory is that when we exercise, our cardiovascular system redistributes blood so that it sends more to our working muscles and less to other areas, such as the gut. This slows digestion and the food sits in the gut for longer, allowing greater absorption of the allergenic protein and triggering a reaction.

We will see a patient with FDEIA in my clinic on average once or twice a month, and it is another allergic condition where allergists turn into detectives to try and find out what is going on. In my clinic it is wheat, and not shellfish, that is the most common culprit food, but many different foods have been reported to cause FDEIA, including tomatoes, eggs and milk.[4]

While someone will usually have to eat a substantial amount of the offending food to cause a reaction, exercise does not always have to be intense: running for a train, or even dancing at a party, may be all it takes to trigger a reaction. In some patients, taking NSAIDs such as ibuprofen can substitute for exercise.

Case study: Sarah

In one particularly memorable case, fifty-four-year-old Sarah was referred to me with 'New Year's Eve allergy'.

For 364 days a year Sarah was fit and well, but she ended up in hospital with severe anaphylaxis on 31 December three years in a row. Unsurprisingly she was starting to dread the New Year festivities.

After talking to Sarah, it became clear that each New Year's Eve had three key things in common: a prawn-cocktail starter was a New Year's Eve tradition; Sarah indulged in a few drinks to see in the New Year; and she loved to dance the night away. Separately she could eat prawns, drink alcohol and exercise (dance) and experience no problems, but the three elements combined spelled trouble.

How is FDEIA diagnosed?

A detailed medical history is needed, and the diagnosis is usually confirmed using skin-prick and blood tests (in the case of FDEIA to wheat, specific IgE to a protein in wheat called omega-5-gliadin will usually be raised). People will generally react within two hours of eating the food, but in some patients it can take much longer. This is why, once we confirm the diagnosis, we advise patients to wait at least four hours before eating the food and exercising.

Tick bites and allergic reactions to red meat

For many people, steak and chips is their idea of a delicious meal, but for some this could spell disaster. In the last twenty years allergy to red meat and offal has emerged as a problem in many parts of the world. And it is all down to ticks – small insects that feed on the blood of animals (including humans). Ticks are best known for causing diseases such as Lyme disease, but they also play a role in one of the most fascinating recent developments in food allergy: alpha-gal syndrome, also known as mammalian meat allergy.

Alpha-gal exists naturally inside all mammals, except for two-legged mammals like chimpanzees and humans. Usually alpha-gal passes through the digestive system and is 'ignored' by our immune system. However, some people who are exposed to alpha-gal through the skin from repeated tick bites may produce IgE antibodies to alpha-gal. They then start to develop allergic reactions, which are often severe, whenever they consume red meat. Inexplicably, this reaction is usually delayed by between two and six hours, but reactions can also occur within minutes or even up to twenty-four hours later. Poultry does not contain alpha-gal, and alpha-gal-allergic patients can continue to eat chicken, turkey and duck. However, for some patients, milk, cheese and gelatin will be problematic.

Alpha-gal is a sugar and, as we know from the previous chapter, food allergies are triggered by proteins, so the emergence of an allergy where patients were reacting to a carbohydrate stunned the allergy world.

Allergy to alpha-gal has been widely described in South and Central American states and Australia. Cases are also reported across Europe, less frequently. Ticks are becoming increasingly common; and in April 2021 the first series of three patients with allergy to alpha-gal in the UK was published.[5]

If you want to know more about tick-bite prevention, a really helpful resource is the CDC website.[6]

How is alpha-gal allergy diagnosed?

Again diagnosis requires a meticulous medical history, followed by skin-prick and blood tests.

A new 'allergy': lipid transfer protein allergy

The mantra of eating five portions of fruit and veg a day has become part of our collective psyche. In addition, more of us are moving to a plant-based diet, and this trend has coincided with the emergence of a new, more severe form of allergy called lipid transfer protein (LTP) allergy – named after the type of proteins in fruits, vegetables, nuts, seeds and cereals that cause a reaction. LTPs are found in all fruit, nuts, seeds and vegetables, with the highest concentrations being found in the peel and pips of plant foods. Common trigger foods include stoned fruit, apples, tomatoes and nuts such as hazelnuts, almonds and walnuts.

LTP allergy was first identified and is widely described in the Mediterranean, but in recent years we have been seeing more LTP-sensitized patients in the UK. And like many things, once you look for it, you find more and more affected patients. Unlike with PFS, patients allergic to LTP will react to both cooked and raw fruits, vegetables and nuts but not always. Another characteristic of this new allergy is that reactions appear to be very much dependent on co-factors such as exercise, alcohol or the ingestion of NSAIDs. It is believed that somehow these co-factors enhance the absorption of the food. So once again these reactions can be hard to diagnose, and the allergist has to turn detective. For allergists, making the diagnosis and solving the puzzle is highly satisfying, resulting in many delighted patients who finally have an answer to the mystery of their allergic reactions.

What is behind this rise in cases? The exact reason is not yet known. Theories abound, but the one with the most evidence is that patients become sensitized to LTP found in tree and weed pollens, and subsequently react when they eat a fruit or vegetable containing LTP.[7]

How is LTP allergy diagnosed?

As always, the first stage is a detailed history; in cases of complex food allergy, don't be surprised if your allergist spends considerable time detailing the reaction and the circumstances around it. If LTP allergy is suspected, there are some nifty blood tests called component allergen tests, that can be checked. These measure specific IgE to the different allergenic proteins in a food. An allergist can thus measure specific IgE to LTP in a range of fruits and nuts and, when this is combined with relevant skin tests, can confirm the diagnosis and give you personalized advice.

8. Delayed Food Allergies

If I were to canvass social media for one word to sum up an allergic reaction, I'd wager most people would offer terms like 'rapid' or 'instant'. But as I mentioned in Chapter 1, allergic reactions are not always due to specific IgE to an allergen. They can involve other parts of the immune system.

These are known as non-IgE-mediated allergies; they are rarer and, because reactions are slower, they are also often described as delayed food allergies. Anaphylaxis is not a feature, adrenaline does not help and they can be much harder to diagnose. In this chapter I will look at three delayed food allergies: delayed cow's milk protein allergy (CMPA), and the much rarer but important conditions of eosinophilic oesophagitis (EoE, see page 96) and food protein-induced enterocolitis syndrome (FPIES, see page 98).

Delayed cow's milk protein allergy

An estimated 1 per cent of babies suffer from CMPA, where symptoms typically begin several hours or even days after having cow's milk. Diagnosis is tricky, because many symptoms overlap with those of other illnesses or conditions that are common in babies, such as vomiting, colic, reflux, constipation, diarrhoea, food refusal and generally being a bit 'snuffly'. These vague general symptoms, combined with industry promotion of formula milks, has led some paediatricians to conclude that this is why the demand for specialist milk formula has sky-rocketed several-fold, in excess of the amount needed for the 1 per cent of infants with CMPA.[1]

In addition, as symptoms are generalized, parents will often report a delay before diagnosis; there are no allergy tests that your family doctor can perform to confirm the diagnosis.

If you are reading this and suspect that your baby has delayed CMPA, you need to be asking the three questions shown on the chart opposite. It is also worth pointing out that weight loss is not a common symptom of delayed CMPA.

If your family doctor or paediatrician agrees that delayed CMPA is a possibility, then your baby should be moved on to a dairy-free diet. If the child is being breastfed, this means the mother will have to cut out dairy from her diet (she should take vitamin D and calcium supplements while doing this). If the child is formula-fed, there are specialist milks for children with CMPA. It is then **essential** to reintroduce dairy products two to four weeks later, to confirm or discount the diagnosis – otherwise you will never know if any improvement in symptoms during the trial is down to cutting out dairy or simply coincidence.

Another, rarer type of delayed CMPA is cow's milk protein-induced proctocolitis. This condition often manifests when a baby is about two months of age, and blood is seen in the nappy of an otherwise-healthy child. It is more common in breastfed babies and usually clears quickly when the mother switches to a dairy-free diet.

The good news is that delayed CMPA is usually out-grown by the time babies reach twelve months of age, and

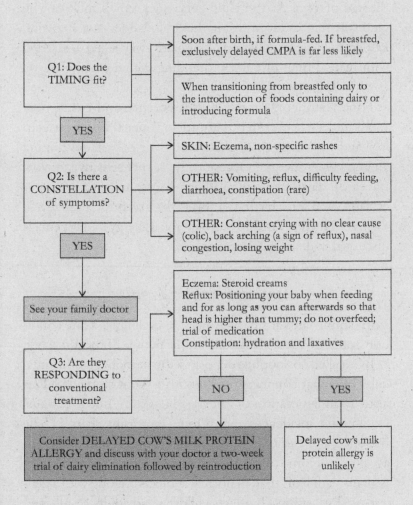

Q1: Does the TIMING fit?

Soon after birth, if formula-fed. If breastfed, exclusively delayed CMPA is far less likely

When transitioning from breastfed only to the introduction of foods containing dairy or introducing formula

YES

Q2: Is there a CONSTELLATION of symptoms?

SKIN: Eczema, non-specific rashes

OTHER: Vomiting, reflux, difficulty feeding, diarrhoea, constipation (rare)

OTHER: Constant crying with no clear cause (colic), back arching (a sign of reflux), nasal congestion, losing weight

YES

See your family doctor

Eczema: Steroid creams
Reflux: Positioning your baby when feeding and for as long as you can afterwards so that head is higher than tummy; do not overfeed; trial of medication
Constipation: hydration and laxatives

Q3: Are they RESPONDING to conventional treatment?

NO

YES

Consider DELAYED COW'S MILK PROTEIN ALLERGY and discuss with your doctor a two-week trial of dairy elimination followed by reintroduction

Delayed cow's milk protein allergy is unlikely

Could it be delayed cow's milk protein allergy (CMPA)?
Three key questions to ask

cow's milk protein-induced proctocolitis usually resolves by the age of two. As the child gets older, cow's milk can be gradually reintroduced, using the 'milk ladder' – a stepwise, graded milk reintroduction. There are twelve steps, starting with malted-milk biscuits and ending with a small glass of cow's milk.

Food allergy only rarely causes eczema, and cutting out foods unnecessarily can be harmful to yourself (if breastfeeding) and your baby (it may increase their risk of developing an immediate allergy). Occasionally, in very sensitive infants, traces of dairy in their mother's breast milk may trigger eczema soon after birth, but this is the exception rather than the rule. The relationship between food allergy and eczema is discussed in detail in Chapter 14.

Eosinophilic oesophagitis

EoE (abbreviated from the American spelling) is a rare condition, more frequently found in atopic people.[2] It occurs when WBCs called eosinophils deposit in the oesophagus, the muscular tube that connects your mouth to your stomach.[3] This leads to inflammation of the oesophagus. While it remains uncommon, incidences appear to be increasing sharply.[4] The reasons are unclear, but may reflect alterations in the oesophageal microbiome (more oesophageal bacteria were found in patients with EoE than in normal subjects[5]), along with a genetic predisposition.[6] It affects children and adults of all ages, with males being three times more likely to develop it.[7]

Patients present with a range of different symptoms, including:

- **Infants and toddlers**: Vomiting, regurgitation, reflux, poor growth and feeding refusal
- **Older children**: Reflux, vomiting or abdominal pain
- **Adolescents and adults**: Reflux, difficulty swallowing and food 'sticking' on the way down the oesophagus.

Common foods that trigger symptoms include milk, egg, wheat and soya – but it's not always the foods that 'stick on the way down' that are the problem.

Again the range of symptoms and the crossover with other conditions means that diagnosis can be tricky, but crucial: EoE is a chronic lifelong condition that can lead to damage in the oesophagus if left untreated.

An Italian study identified an average three-year delay between first symptoms appearing and getting a diagnosis,[8] while a Danish study found there was a ten-year delay in making the diagnosis.[9] It is likely that this delay in diagnosis reflects a lack of knowledge both among family doctors and among gastroenterologists. In addition people with EoE seem remarkably able to cope, but when I have told patients in my clinic what I suspect is happening, and that I have a name for their condition, I have felt their palpable relief.

If EoE is suspected, patients are prescribed a six-week course of medication called a proton-pump inhibitor, which blocks stomach acid, to see if their symptoms improve. If they do, their symptoms are not due to EoE, but to acid reflux. If the symptoms persist and EoE is suspected, a diagnosis is made by taking a biopsy of the oesophagus and measuring the number of eosinophils.

Treatment generally involves using a steroid inhaler to reduce inflammation and eliminating multiple food groups, then reintroducing them under allergy-dietician supervision. In the future the new biologic drug dupilumab (see pages 187–8) may also be an option, with early data showing that it suppresses the oesophageal inflammation seen in EoE.[10]

Food protein-induced enterocolitis syndrome

FPIES is a rare but serious condition in children, where delayed food allergy – most commonly due to milk or soya – triggers severe inflammation in the gut. About one to four hours after ingesting the food the child develops severe vomiting and lethargy, and sometimes diarrhoea. A serious reaction can lead to a loss of fluids and shock, and many children will end up in A&E.

If your child has repeated episodes of vomiting, keep a detailed food diary and discuss this with your family doctor. If FPIES is suspected, paediatric input is essential. Depending on where you live, this may be a general paediatrician, a paediatric gastroenterologist or a paediatric allergist. Symptoms resolve when the offending foods are eliminated. Fortunately this is a condition that children appear to grow out of, and 90 per cent of children will usually find that FPIES clears up between the ages of three and five years.[11]

9: How Will I Cope? – Living with a Food Allergy

The smell of your mum's cooking, childhood birthday parties, celebratory meals to remember and the culinary disasters to forget – food plays such a central part of our lives. But when you live with a food allergy, so much of that enjoyment can be hampered. Many patients and their families describe struggling to be taken seriously, and this is compounded by the stress of everyday events – such as the supermarket shop, going out for a meal, picking up a quick snack or catching a flight – triggering anxiety that one wrong move will result in a reaction.

Your allergies can be a hurdle, of course, but they should never be a barrier to you leading a full and happy life. In this chapter I will be helping you navigate everyday events: from the information you can expect when eating in a restaurant or ordering a takeaway, to making sure that your airline is allergy-aware. I will be giving you some simple strategies and checklists to make sure that you are prepared, and to make the experience as stress-free as possible.

I will also be looking at those milestone moments when food plays such a central part, including starting school and attending children's birthday parties. And I will discuss how young people can educate their peers about their allergies, when starting university or moving away from home for the first time.

Eating out with a food allergy

The main message here is that of course you can enjoy a meal out with friends or loved ones, but you need to exercise some caution and do your homework before you dine out.

Seven top tips for enjoying eating out

1. Have your medication with you and make certain it is in date. Ensure that those with you know what to do, if you react.
2. Always check the ingredients in a dish, even if you have eaten it before – recipes may change, and chefs can alter recipes!
3. Do your homework: half of the fun of eating out is opening the menu and choosing what to eat, but this can be stressful with a food allergy. Book ahead where possible, check the menu online and, if you have any questions, call before your visit.
4. Book your table wisely: a Saturday night at 8p.m. or a pre-theatre meal in the heart of London's West End, when restaurants are full and staff are crazy busy, may not be the best time to choose. If you don't have much room for manoeuvre over timing – for example, on a special group outing or a work trip – call the restaurant at a quieter time to discuss your allergy.
5. Ask questions: be polite but assertive. *Can I see your allergen information? How do you take*

allergens into account when preparing food? If you feel you aren't getting the level of detail you need, ask to speak to a manager.

6. Trust your gut: if you don't feel comfortable about the surroundings or confident in the information given to you by the staff, leave. Find somewhere else that you do feel confident will cater to your needs. It's really not worth taking the risk.

7. If you are going abroad, consider getting a food-allergy translation card (see Further Reading and Resources on page 221).

Fourteen food allergens

According to European Union law, food businesses must declare if any of the fourteen allergens shown overleaf (see the illustration) – which have been identified as the most potent and prevalent food allergens – are used in any food they sell or provide. This law has been retained post-Brexit and, according to the UK's Food Standards Agency, when eating out or ordering a takeaway the restaurant or café must provide you with allergen information in writing. This could be via allergen information printed on the menu or a prompt explaining how to obtain allergen information, such as speaking to a member of staff.[1] The way this information is provided depends on the type of food you buy and the sort of food business you are buying it from.[2]

(Tip: if you are reading this book elsewhere in the world, check the website of your food-standards authority to see if a similar scheme is in operation.)

Celery

Cereals containing
gluten (such as
barley and oats)

Crustaceans
(such as prawns,
crab and lobster)

Eggs

Fish

Lupin
(legume belonging to
the same plant family
as peanuts)

Milk

Molluscs
(such as mussels
and oysters)

Mustard

Peanuts

Sesame

Soya beans

Sulphites
(at a concentration
of more than ten
parts per million)

Tree nuts
(such as almonds,
hazelnuts, walnuts,
Brazil nuts, cashews,
pecans, pistachios and
macadamia nuts)

Fourteen food allergens

<u>Get yourself a medical-alert bracelet, not a tattoo</u>
A medical-alert bracelet is worn on the wrist and
carries details of your health conditions, medication
or allergies. There are lots of options available
online, and it is something that I would recommend
is worn by anyone with a confirmed food, venom or
drug allergy, in case you cannot communicate your
allergies for any reason. There has been a trend in
recent years for medical tattoos, but these are not the
same! Medical professionals may not see them and,
even if they do, they will not be sure whether or not
to take them seriously.

In addition, if you have a letter from an allergist,
keep a copy with you, or a screenshot on your phone,
so that you have it to hand.

Food shopping and eating on the go

Under UK food law, if any of the fourteen allergens listed
above are present in food, they must be 'emphasized' or easy
to spot on the list of ingredients on the label – for example,
written in bold or italic type. (Again, if you are reading this in
another country, check local food-labelling laws – Australia,
for instance, has a similar system in place to the UK.)

How do I spot allergens on pre-packed food?

Tragically, in July 2016 fifteen-year-old Natasha Ednan-
Laperouse died of anaphylaxis on a flight from London to
France, after eating sesame in an artichoke, olive and tapenade

baguette bought in an airport sandwich shop. The case hit the headlines, and her parents have since campaigned tirelessly for a change in UK food laws, to afford the protection to others that they so sorely lacked. On 1 October 2021 'Natasha's Law', which requires food businesses to include full ingredient labelling on every food item 'pre-packed for direct sale' (PPDS), came into force.[3]

Examples of PPDS that now require labelling include:

- Sandwiches and bakery products packed onsite before a customer selects or orders them
- Products pre-packaged onsite ready for sale, such as pizzas, rotisserie chicken, salads and pasta pots
- Burgers and sausages pre-packaged by a butcher on the premises, ready for sale to consumers
- Foods packaged and then sold elsewhere by the same operator at a market stall or mobile site
- PPDS food provided in schools, care homes or hospitals.

Non pre-packed (loose) food

Food businesses such as bakeries or delicatessens must provide you with allergen information for any loose item you buy that contains any of the fourteen allergens. But loose food – be it street food or food from a market stall, buffet or popcorn in a cinema – has an intrinsically higher risk of cross-contamination. It is best to avoid it if possible.

Remember: If you are allergic to ingredients that are not among the fourteen allergens, always check the label or ask staff for more details.

Always check the label – and check behind the label, too

Tanya Wright is an allergy specialist dietician and author who has first-hand experience of living with food allergy. She says: 'It is very important that you avoid foods or derivatives of foods that you are allergic to. If there is a label on the product, you will be able to check the ingredients; however, it is important that you know what it is you are checking for, and that you understand all the names for the food you are allergic to. For example, broad bean and fava bean are the same thing. Always avoid foods that do not have a label, or you will not know the ingredients. Do not take a risk by guessing if it is safe or not. Foods with precautionary labelling can be a risk for those who react to trace allergens. This labelling can be under many guises – for example, "made in a factory using . . .", "may contain traces of . . ." If you are not carrying allergy rescue medications, or you are away from medical help, you should not consume these foods even if you have had them before. If you have reacted to trace amounts in the past, you should always avoid foods with precautionary labelling.'

Be warned: in some countries, labels may peel back and there may be more ingredients listed **behind** the first label. So always check.

Flying with food allergies

Flying can be stressful at the best of times, but there is an understandable added layer of anxiety with a food allergy. This is compounded by different airlines having different policies in place. Again preparation is your friend and, from booking to boarding, your food allergy should be front and centre of your mind at all times when flying.

- Make sure you declare your own (or your child's) allergies with your travel-insurance company in case you need to make a claim while you are away.
- Check your airline's allergy policy –including connecting flights, which may be with a different carrier. The UK charity Anaphylaxis Campaign has a helpful page with the allergy policies of several airlines.[4]
- If you are taking lots of allergy-friendly food for your holiday, check if your airline will give you excess luggage allowance. Some will, on receipt of a signed letter from your doctor.
- Food for the flight: ask when booking if an allergy-free meal can be ordered, or bring your own food for the journey.
- Signpost your allergy at every opportunity – including when booking your flight, at check-in, when boarding and when food and drink are served in the air.
- Be allergy-aware as soon as you step in the airport, including in airport lounges, bars and restaurants. Arrive early to find a suitable place to buy food and drink, giving you time to read the labels and ask questions of staff.
- Check, check and triple-check that you have adequate medication in your hand luggage for the flight. Is your AAI in date? Are you wearing your medical-alert bracelet? Ensure that all medication is within reach for the flight, such as in the seat pocket, and not stowed away in an overhead locker.

- Bring a packet of wipes to wipe down your seat, armrest and tray table once you have boarded.

Keeping your child safe at school

I am constantly in awe of how my patients and families manage food allergies, and the time, care and effort that go into creating an allergy-safe environment. So it is entirely understandable that a milestone like a first day at school can be daunting for parents of children who are living with food allergies.

In the UK schools have a legal duty to support pupils at their school with medical conditions, including allergies.[5] All pupils with a medical condition have in place a document called an Individual Healthcare Plan (IHP). Agreed between parents and the school, this document includes:

- Details of your child's condition and symptoms
- Daily requirements, including medication such as an auto-injector device and any dietary needs
- Who will administer medication
- Action to take in the event of a medical emergency
- Contact details for the next of kin, family doctor and sometimes the child's allergy specialist.

How can I, as a parent, help my child's school to be more allergy-safe?

The last thing any parent wants is for their child to be unsafe, or even at risk of being picked on because of a lack of knowledge concerning their allergies. Your school will have a legal responsibility for your child's safety, but there are steps you can take to help raise awareness and change mindsets.

- **How allergy-aware is your child's school?** The charity Allergy UK has an online test where families can check if their child's school is allergy-aware. It covers whether a school (currently only secondary schools) has a medicines-management policy and a food-allergy policy.[6]
- **Encourage children to talk about their allergies**. I'm not suggesting that they bring their AAI to their next show-and-tell, but classmates may be curious and will ask questions. Being open and honest about your child's allergy will help to normalize their condition.
- **Suggest some whole-school education on allergies** – teachers and students included. For younger children, this could start with a storybook about allergies at story-time. A good one is *Luca . . . the Lion Who Couldn't Eat Meat* by Tersha Cutmore – a great little book, beautifully illustrated, which conveys an important message about difference and allergy awareness.

From parties to play dates: navigating social occasions when your child has an allergy

Allergies can be incredibly isolating, especially for younger children, and play dates and parties can be an important way of bringing some fun and friendship into your child's life. Here are some tips on navigating that tricky path between keeping your child safe and well and letting him or her form important social bonds and memories. The main thing I would advise is never, ever to be afraid of talking about your child's allergies. You aren't being fussy, or a 'helicopter' parent. You are simply looking out for your child and imparting important information, as any parent in your shoes would do.

- **Be clear and concise about your child's allergies**. It is much more common nowadays for parents to ask ahead of a party or play date if children have any allergies. Be specific in your answer and make sure all the key information is covered. Put yourself in their shoes: what do they need to know? What are your child's allergies, what are the symptoms of an allergic reaction, what medication do they need, plus what to do in an emergency.
- **Put it in writing**. Allergy information could be communicated verbally on the phone or at the school gate, but always follow it up in writing, such as in a friendly text or even by adapting the sample letter below; attach the child's anaphylaxis management plan (if they have one from their specialist) and pop it in your child's bag.

> **<u>Sample letter for parents</u>**
> **Dear [*insert name*]**
> **<u>Notification of [*insert allergy or allergies*] in</u>**
> **[*insert child's name – put this information in large, underlined bold type*]**
> **My child has an allergy to [*insert details*]**
> **The symptoms of an allergic reaction are [*insert details*]**
> **They require [*list any medication they take*]**

In the event of an emergency [*include any specific actions to take*]

I would request that this letter is circulated among current staff and/or volunteers and is shown to all new members of staff in future.

If you have any questions, please contact me on [*include your name, phone number and email address*].

- **Any questions?** It can be daunting for another parent (or even a family member) to care for your child. If you sense they are unsure, remind them that they can ask you anything and everything to make the event as smooth and enjoyable for your child as possible.
- **Talk to children** about what to do if they have a reaction. Make sure you are clear about how an allergic reaction may feel, and the need to tell an appointed grown-up immediately if they start to feel unwell.
- **Provide your own snacks**, if in doubt.

Most childcare settings these days will insist on any birthday cakes being shop-bought so that it is easy to identify the ingredients. But parties and play dates will often rely on homemade sandwiches and treats, which might not be so easy to keep track of.

I always remember a story from a (now grown-up) patient of mine, who has CMPA. Every year his family would go to the coast for their summer holidays, but when the time came for ice-cream on the beach, he would watch his siblings devouring huge ice-creams while he had to make do with a dry, empty ice-cream cone to chew on.

Packing a little lunchbox full of your child's favourite snacks or treats will ensure they don't miss out on any of the fun.

Striking out on your own: a guide for young adults with food allergy

Starting university or moving out of home for the first time is a hugely exciting time: new friends, new surroundings . . . and new challenges when it comes to your food allergies.

Case study: Archie

Archie was two when he was diagnosed with CMPA. Throughout his childhood his parents faced the usual challenge of explaining his allergy to family and friends, some of whom were less understanding than others – particularly one well-meaning aunt who insisted that he was only a 'little bit allergic' and that skimmed milk surely wouldn't hurt him. Then came the play dates and parties: worries about whether Archie could eat the food and whether the food was safe to eat, and tears when birthday cake was off-limits. Archie's mum, Claire, would feel a familiar knot in her stomach when dropping him off at a play date, even with close friends.

As Archie reached his teenage years, things began to get easier. A naturally shy boy, he slowly grew in confidence in talking about his allergy. He was aware of his triggers and recognized the signs of an allergic reaction. One big positive was when Archie started secondary school, where his parents both worked as teachers. It meant that keeping staff and classmates informed about his allergy was more straightforward.

Archie worked hard through his teenage years and won a place to read economics at university. However, the only sticking point was that the university was a two-hour drive away from home. Claire said she felt the familiar knot in her stomach return: having to explain his allergy to new friends, and the dangers of cross-contamination in a shared kitchen in his hall of residence. Luckily Archie took it all in his stride. With his new-found confidence, he was clear about his allergy when meeting his new housemates, kept his food in a repurposed beer fridge and staggered cooking times in the kitchen, to avoid cross-contamination.

'Everyone was really understanding,' says Archie, now twenty. 'My allergy always made me feel a bit "different". But now I'm in an environment where being different is a good thing, so I've kind of embraced it.'

At home you will no doubt have developed your own routines and coping strategies, and your nearest and dearest will know all about your allergies. But in new surroundings, such as university halls of residence, and on nights out in new places, it can be easy for things to go awry.

- **If starting university**, make staff aware of your allergies. This includes tutors, administrative staff and catering staff, if you have a meal plan.
- **Be upfront** with new friends and housemates. Never feel embarrassed about disclosing your condition. Try jotting down a few notes on your phone to remind you of the key things you need to communicate.
- **If you use an autoinjector,** bring a trainer pen and let your new flatmates or friends try it out.
- **Don't forget your phone**. Keep it charged and topped up, in case of emergency, and change your lock screen to a message stating that you have a food allergy.
- **Eating out or drinking in a new place?** Check the menu ahead of your visit, and ask staff questions about the ingredients in food and drink. Cocktails, smoothies and juices are best avoided as they can be a hidden source of allergens. If you are unsure – don't risk it.
- **Going on a date?** If you plan on a kiss, be allergen-aware: make sure your date hasn't eaten any food containing your allergen for at least four hours prior to locking lips.
- **Think pockets!** Is there somewhere to store your adrenaline pen? Are you wearing a medical-alert bracelet?
- **Sharing a kitchen?** Keep your utensils separate, your sponge for washing your dishes separate and stay out of the kitchen if allergens are around. If you can afford it and there is space, have your own fridge or own shelf in the fridge (the top shelf, to prevent others' foods dropping onto yours). Ideally you should be the first person in the kitchen in the morning and evening, so that you can use the space ahead of others, to prevent

cross-contamination. If eating as a group, there should be an allergen-free option, and it is safest if you prepare it yourself. Ask your flatmates to let you know if they are going to be cooking with something that you are allergic to.

10. Anaphylaxis: Reducing the Fear – What You Should Know

Case study: Emily

One afternoon, while I was writing the rhinitis chapter for this book, a friend called me. I first met Kate when she interviewed me for an article about allergy for a national newspaper, and we hit it off and became friends. She has a beautiful daughter, Emily, a lively six-year-old who loves helping her mum in the garden and stoically navigates her way through life with allergies to egg, nuts, sesame and wheat.

During the phone call Kate's usual bubbly voice was strained: Emily was having an allergic reaction. One of the mums who splits the school-run duties with Kate gave Emily some chocolate as an after-school treat. She took it from a multipack, and while the ingredients were listed on the outside of the packet, they weren't given on each individual chocolate, so she hadn't clocked that it contained egg-white powder. Emily had developed tummy ache soon afterwards, but nobody had realized this could herald the start of an anaphylactic reaction.

'Emily is home now, has a rash and says she feels "itchy",' Kate explained to me. 'I have given her some antihistamine, but should I use our adrenaline pen? She doesn't look distressed, she is watching Netflix. She isn't wheezing and her tummy pain is settling. I'm probably making a fuss . . .'

If Kate was on the point of questioning whether or not to give adrenaline, that usually meant it was needed – and fast. 'I can hear Emily coughing continuously, and it means her airways are irritated,' I told Kate. 'I want you to get her EpiPen and inject her in her upper thigh. Don't feel nervous about it. Give it to her now and I'll call you back.' I then hung up to give Kate time to put my advice into action.

I called Kate back ten minutes later. Thankfully Emily had responded to the adrenaline and was much better. The coughing had stopped, and they were waiting for an ambulance to take her to hospital for observation. I felt relieved and thought Kate's usual upbeat voice had returned. But then suddenly I heard her voice crumple. She was crying.

'I kept thinking: it will be fine – we've got the EpiPen, we've got Sophie on the phone. But at the same time I had this other stream of thought: I was thinking about the headlines and all the stories. I didn't want us to be the next tragic case study, seated on the sofa and talking to the news. I kept thinking that it happened so fast and we knew what to do, but what happens if Emily is in a scenario where she is surrounded by people who don't know what to do? She is going to have to live with this for the rest of her life. I feel scared of the present. I feel scared for the future.'

My heart melted as she told me this. 'Kate, you thought you'd found your balance of managing this, but this has just upended it all. We love our children and it's natural to have these emotions. It would be more surprising if you did not feel this way. You just need time to process it all and then work out your new balance. For the moment, the main thing is that Emily is fine. You have done all the right things, and I just want you to focus on her. Let's chat again soon and, if you are worried, call me anytime.'

An introduction to anaphylaxis

Anaphylactic (pronounced 'anna-fill-actic') reactions are severe allergic reactions that are usually due to food, drug or venom allergy. The first recorded case may have been as early as 2641 BCE, when the pharaoh Menes succumbed to a wasp sting.

Nowadays, food is the most likely trigger of an anaphylactic reaction requiring hospital admission to hospital, but the most common cause of fatal reactions are drugs.[1] In my experience, the most severe anaphylactic reactions are in those who are allergic to general-anaesthetic agents or who react to bee and wasp stings. In people who are allergic to stings, they are receiving an injection of the allergen directly into the muscle, so reactions can be very quick. In addition they may be outdoors and far from help.

However, I am all too aware that the group of patients

whose quality of life is the most impacted by the risk of anaphylaxis are those with food allergy. Food is a social lubricant, it is a way that we connect and socialize and often it means pleasure. However, living with a food allergy can mean that daily tasks such as going shopping, eating out or, in Emily's case, something as simple as a child being given chocolate as a treat is fraught with stress and the anxiety of potential complication (see Chapter 9 for tips about living with a food allergy). When I spoke to Kate later, she told me that she did not want to come across as a super-stressed parent and insist that Emily's pick-up had a set of AAIs for a ten-minute journey home. That has now changed; she finds it easier to be assertive and wherever Emily goes, her AAIs go with her.

As an allergist I have seen thousands of patients who have experienced severe allergic reactions or anaphylaxis. I have taught doctors, nurses and pharmacists about anaphylaxis management, both in the UK and abroad. I have spoken about anaphylaxis on social media, in the written press, on the radio and on TV, and I have recently been consulted on the Resuscitation Council UK's anaphylaxis guidelines. Most importantly, my patients have taught me through their life experiences and lived knowledge of anaphylaxis.

In this chapter I want to share with you my experience of looking after patients with anaphylaxis, and give you lots of practical tips to help keep you or your loved ones safe. Tragically, more than half of those dying from anaphylaxis to foods in the UK have had no professional advice about their food allergy.[2] So if you are unsure whether you are at risk of anaphylaxis, please talk to your family doctor, who should be able to refer you, if appropriate, to an allergy specialist. And if you have had an anaphylactic reaction and are waiting to be seen by an allergy clinic, ask your family doctor to prescribe you an AAI. Waits for appointments in some countries can be long, and you want to be able to treat yourself in case of further reaction. In addition, if you are carrying adrenaline and have never been under the care of a specialist clinic, ask your family doctor to refer you, in order that your allergies can be confirmed and your management plan reviewed.

Symptoms of anaphylaxis

Anaphylaxis usually begins within minutes of exposure to an allergen and usually progresses fast. Allergic reactions cross over into anaphylaxis if they affect a person's breathing or they cause a person's blood pressure to drop and can lead to the lungs failing (respiratory failure) or the heart suddenly stopping (cardiac arrest).

Other symptoms may include itchy skin, hives, facial swelling, an itchy mouth, nausea and vomiting, abdominal pain or a congested nose. But it is important to point out none of these symptoms by themselves make a diagnosis of anaphylaxis.

In the case of an anaphylactic reaction to foods, the main symptoms are usually linked to the airway or breathing difficulties (see the illustration overleaf). So if someone with a known food allergy – or even you yourself – suddenly starts coughing or wheezing during or shortly after eating, ask yourself: Could it be anaphylaxis?

Anaphylactic reactions to stings and drugs usually present with a drop in blood pressure. Signs of low blood pressure include feeling dizzy, light-headed, faint, becoming clammy

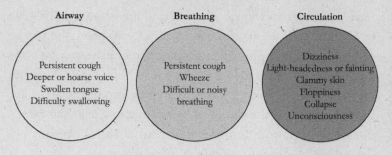

The ABC of anaphylaxis symptoms

and generally being less 'with it'. If a reaction is very severe, then both difficulty in breathing and signs of low blood pressure may be present.

> **<u>Top tip: don't believe everything you see on TV</u>**
> Although no less worrying, anaphylaxis does not have to be dramatic, as it is commonly shown in films and on medical dramas – the symptoms fall in a spectrum of severity. A rash and a cough, like Emily experienced, is anaphylaxis. Facial swelling and collapsing minutes after a wasp sting also counts as anaphylaxis. Regardless of severity, if you are thinking anaphylaxis, then adrenaline is the treatment of choice. Do not lose precious time taking antihistamines and 'waiting to see' what happens. Antihistamines do not treat anaphylaxis.

How quickly will an anaphylactic reaction occur?

Timing is critical when diagnosing anaphylaxis:

- Almost all anaphylactic reactions to food will occur within thirty minutes of eating the allergen. Reactions hardly ever occur more than two hours later.
- Anaphylaxis to bee and wasp stings usually occurs within a few minutes of being stung and rarely more than thirty minutes later.
- Anaphylaxis to tablet medication usually occurs within thirty minutes, although reactions can be far quicker (minutes) if the medication is injected.

Treatment: adrenaline

The only proven way to stop anaphylaxis is with a shot of adrenaline – antihistamines simply won't cut it in these situations. Adrenaline is effective for all symptoms of anaphylaxis. It is safe. It acts rapidly. It works by quickly opening up the airways, reducing swelling and increasing blood pressure.

Most people with a severe food or sting allergy will be prescribed an AAI (in Emily's case, a chunky pen-sized device called an EpiPen), which is pre-filled with adrenaline to use in an emergency. Yet, staggeringly, a study by Canadian allergist Professor Estelle Simons found that about one-third of people prescribed adrenaline by their doctor do not take their prescription to a chemist and get their AAI.[3]

Please, please don't be one of them. Equally, if you already have an autoinjector, put this book down and go and check it is still in date. If it is out of date, call your doctor today for a new one. While using an out-of-date auto-injector in an emergency is unlikely to harm you, it is likely to be less effective. If you have a child with a food allergy, check that you have the correct AAI for your child's weight.

> **<u>Put it in the diary</u>**
> **On the same day you collect your new adrenaline autoinjector, set an alert on your phone or make a note in your diary one month before it is due to expire. This will remind you in good time when you should be asking for a replacement. Some manufacturers also offer a text reminder service: check the patient information leaflet that comes with your autoinjector.**

Why prompt use of adrenaline is vital

In 1992 paediatrician Professor Hugh Sampson published a sobering paper in the *New England Journal of Medicine*. He compared the cases of six children and adolescents who died of anaphylactic reactions to foods with seven others who nearly died. All thirteen children, aged two to seventeen years, had known food allergies, but had unknowingly eaten the foods responsible for the reaction. None of the six who died received adrenaline within thirty minutes, and only two received it within the first hour. In contrast, six of the seven who survived received adrenaline within thirty minutes. The stark conclusion was that prompt administration of adrenaline during anaphylaxis significantly reduces the risk of a fatal outcome.

Dying as a result of an anaphylactic reaction is, thankfully, an incredibly rare event. Anaphylactic reactions do not build up or automatically get progressively worse. However, as nobody can predict whether a reaction will become life-threatening or settle down, the prompt use of adrenaline is always recommended.

Yet numerous studies across the world continue to show the underuse of adrenaline. A UK study found that only 17 per cent of children had been administered an autoinjector when experiencing anaphylaxis.[4] There are many reasons for this, including a lack of training to recognize a severe reaction, a fear of injection or just not having the AAI to hand.[5] Nonetheless, it is worrying, as most cases of fatal and near-fatal anaphylaxis are associated with delayed adrenaline administration.

So if you suspect anaphylaxis, **don't delay** – it is better to use your AAI and then find out it was a false alarm rather than waiting too late. Remember, antihistamines won't cut it; they will not reverse anaphylaxis – they are not designed for that – they will simply treat itchy skin and hives. Also make sure your child knows what to do if they have an allergic reaction, as well as babysitters and family members. To have the best chance of reversing anaphylaxis, adrenaline must be given as soon as possible if there are any signs of airway or breathing difficulties or low blood pressure, even if seemingly mild.

Using an adrenaline pen in the case of a false alarm, or even by accident, won't cause harm. We all have adrenaline circulating around our body. Side-effects of administering an AAI (if any) are mild and may include feeling a bit jittery or your heart racing for a short time. Used or expired AAI should be disposed off at your doctor's surgery, or a hospital or a pharmacy.

Choosing and using an adrenaline autoinjector

As we have seen, the medical term for an adrenaline pen is an adrenaline autoinjector, or AAI. There are different AAIs on the market in different countries, such as the EpiPen, Jext, Auvi-Q and Emerade, but they all require you to self-inject into the middle of your outer thigh. Regardless of the device you are prescribed, there are certain golden rules:

1. **Carry it with you**: Keep your AAI to hand at all times. Dashing up a flight of stairs to a locked bedroom drawer, or running out to the car to fetch it, is the last thing you want to do during an anaphylactic reaction, and the added stress and exertion will probably make your reaction worse. If you doctor has prescribed you more than one autoinjector, then keep both with you and **do not** split them, in case you require a second dose of adrenaline. In my experience, many people are not good at regularly carrying their AAI, but you need to treat them a bit like your mobile phone or house keys and keep them near you. To this end, the UK charity Anaphylaxis Campaign has produced a film encouraging people to carry their adrenaline. If you haven't seen it, it is worth watching, and I often show it to my patients.[6]

2. **Know when to use it**: If you have accidentally eaten something that you are allergic to, or have been stung and are worried about reacting:

- Call for help, so that you are not alone.
- Keep your phone next to you.
- Get your adrenaline pens out, but only use it if you develop signs of anaphylaxis, such as breathing difficulties or indications of low blood pressure.
- It is important to be clear about which symptoms require adrenaline and which do not, so familiarize yourself with the ABC table (see page 120) and teach your close friends, family and even work colleagues, so that they know what to do if you react.
- Remember that an autoinjector will not prevent anaphylaxis before it has occurred, because adrenaline only lasts for a few minutes once it enters the circulation.

3. **Know how to use it**: An adrenaline pen is like an insurance policy – you hope that you never need to use it. But it is crucial that if an emergency does occur, you know how to use it properly. Practice makes perfect. A great way to familiarize yourself with the action and technique is by using a trainer pen. Trainer pens look like the real thing, minus the needle and the adrenaline. Your doctor may be able to give you one, but if not, AAI manufacturers will be able to send you one free of charge and they have step-by-step instructions on how to use it on their websites.[7]

Top tip: practise!
Make sure you use your trainer pen regularly, and be aware that sometimes, due to supply limitations, you may need to switch brands of autoinjector.

If you do, it is essential that you know how to use the new device. When your autoinjector expires, before taking it to a chemist so that it can be safely disposed of, practise firing it into an orange so that you become more familiar with it.

I know the thought of injecting yourself can be daunting. You can train someone else to inject you, but it is imperative that they practise and know what to do. However, it is better if you can inject yourself, as you never know when a reaction may occur. In my experience, patients who have had to use their autoinjectors themselves always say they are glad to have done so, and that it was a lot less scary than they thought it would be. Often they tell me that the experience really boosts their confidence.

Anaphylaxis in focus

Dr Paul Turner, my colleague at St Mary's, carried out a large-scale review of global anaphylaxis admissions. He found evidence of a convincing rise for anaphylaxis across all countries, which was largely due to allergic reactions to medication and food.[8]

For the remainder of this chapter I will be looking in greater detail at the three main causes of anaphylaxis: food allergy, venom allergy and drug allergy. And I will finish with some advice for the family and friends of those with anaphylaxis.

Anaphylaxis to foods

The patients whom I see in my clinic with anaphylaxis to foods tend to fall into two groups:

1. Younger people with food allergy since childhood, who also have rhinitis and asthma.
2. People who develop a new food allergy in adulthood and may not have other allergies.

It is the first group – those with food allergy, rhinitis and asthma – who make up the majority of my patients. Severe reactions are more likely to occur if their asthma is poorly controlled; and if their rhinitis is severe, it can also aggravate their asthma. So managing their anaphylaxis risk involves making sure that their rhinitis and asthma are impeccably controlled.

Is my asthma controlled?
Controlled asthma means:

1. You usually don't have any breathing difficulties, coughing or wheezing.
2. You have few asthma symptoms at night or even after exercise.
3. You can exercise without asthma symptoms.
4. You are not missing work or school because of asthma.
5. You do not need your reliever more than three times a week (apart from when exercising).

If you think, when going through this list, that your asthma is not well controlled, then there could be lots of reasons, including: being exposed to a trigger that is worsening your asthma; not using your preventer inhaler regularly; not using your inhalers in the right way; or not being prescribed the right medication to treat your asthma. So please speak to your family doctor or specialist.

All allergy clinics make a great effort to manage the overall 'allergic burden' of food allergy patients. As well as making sure asthma is well managed, controlling hay fever is particularly relevant, as the risk of food-related anaphylaxis admissions, at least in England, is 22 per cent higher in June compared to January, particularly in children younger than fifteen years.[9]

The second group of patients are more likely to report reactions that are co-factor-dependent – in other words, they will only react to a particular food in the presence of another external factor and may not have the full burden of atopic disease.

Top tip: don't go to the bathroom alone

Often our first instinct, if we feel unwell, is to excuse ourselves and go to the bathroom. However, going there alone is not a good strategy if you think you are suffering an allergic reaction, because they can progress very fast and you may then be alone and unable to get help with terrible consequences. So if you have to go to the bathroom, take someone with you. And make people aware that you are feeling unwell. Never try and manage this alone.

Case study: Lewis

Most severe anaphylactic reactions to foods occur because several risk factors collide, worsening the reaction. Lewis was a nineteen-year-old patient whom I saw several years ago. He was allergic to cow's milk and hen's egg, and he was with friends, eating a wrap that he had bought from a takeaway, when someone grabbed his phone. He ran after the person who had stolen it, but after a few minutes had to stop because he found it hard to breathe.

He had left his adrenaline pens and his blue rescue inhaler behind (they were in his bag) when he ran out of the shop. By the time his friends found him, Lewis was feeling dizzy, wheezing, sweating, nauseous and was covered in hives. He tried to use his rescue asthma inhaler, but it was empty. His friends were not sure how to use his adrenaline pens, and when they realized they were out of date they decided not to administer them. By the time the paramedics arrived, Lewis had almost stopped breathing. He was given multiple doses of adrenaline and was rushed to A&E by ambulance.

I was asked to review Lewis in intensive care. Going through his notes, I could see how the risk factors had layered up, one on top of the other:

1. **Look out for hidden ingredients**: Allergy to cow's milk and eggs can be tricky to manage because they are found in so many foods, and we retrospectively found out that Lewis's takeaway had changed its

recipe, and the grilled chicken had been marinated in buttermilk. There is increasing evidence that in those who do not outgrow their allergy to cow's milk, it is a common cause not only of anaphylaxis, but also of near-fatal and fatal anaphylaxis. In the UK, in school-aged children, cow's milk is now the most common cause of fatal anaphylaxis.[10]

2. **Lewis had eaten the same wrap at the same takeaway before** and therefore presumed the ingredients would be the same. Always check the ingredients if you are eating out, even if you have eaten the same food before. Takeaways and small food outlets may not be as skilled as larger outlets and chains at managing patients with food allergies and can therefore be higher-risk places to eat.

3. **Lewis's hay fever was very badly controlled** and the unchecked inflammation was worsening his asthma. (For more on the 'united airways theory', see page 38.)

4. **Lewis was relying on multiple doses of his rescue inhaler** to help his breathing instead of using a regular preventer. A rescue inhaler does not treat the underlying inflammation that is seen in asthma, so his airways were already twitchy and irritable when he developed anaphylaxis. Needing multiple daily doses of the blue rescue inhaler is a red flag that someone's asthma is uncontrolled.

5. **The exercise would have worsened his reaction** when Lewis ran after the person who had stolen his phone. (For more about co-factors, see Chapter 7.)

6. **Lewis was standing up, despite feeling dizzy.**
Correct posture (either sitting or lying down) is
critical (see below) during anaphylaxis.

7. **There was a delay in the administration of
adrenaline.** This is a common problem. A study
from the Nationwide Children's Hospital in Ohio
found that fewer than 50 per cent of the patients with
a known food allergy had their AAI immediately to
hand at the time of the reaction.[11]

8. **None of Lewis's friends knew what to do** in the
event of a reaction, although they were aware of his
allergy, and none of them knew how to administer
his AAI. Although out of date by a few months,
the AAI could still have been administered and
might have helped. Instead there was panic. It is so
important when you go out that your friends, family
and teammates know how to administer your AAI –
you don't have to do this alone.

Fortunately Lewis left intensive care forty-eight hours
later, unscathed. But I have seen cases go the other way
and it is utterly devastating.

Lie flat, sit or stand?
Fatal anaphylaxis has been associated with standing
up. This is because your blood pressure drops and,
when you stand up, your heart and brain do not
receive an adequate blood supply. No amount of

adrenaline can reverse the effects of gravity, so if you have a history of allergy and start to feel dizzy or light-headed during an anaphylactic reaction, lie flat. If breathing is difficult lying down, then you can sit. Whatever you do, do not suddenly stand up. Very gradually move from lying to sitting and then standing.

<u>Top tip: create an allergy support network</u>
Make sure that family (including grandparents), friends, babysitters, sports coaches and so on – you get my drift – know what to do in cases of anaphylaxis. The last thing you want is for them to be panicking. Teach them – help them to help you. This is not going over the top. Be bold about it. Emergencies are difficult, and this ensures that should an emergency arise, you have the best chance of getting through it unscathed.

Anaphylaxis to bee and wasp stings

It is normal, when you are stung, to develop a painful swelling at the site of the sting. Some people can develop considerable swelling at the site and this is called a large local reaction. Local reactions, while uncomfortable and dramatic-looking, can easily be treated with antihistamines and steroid tablets. However, a very small minority of patients develop a systemic allergic reaction to a sting, so the venom leads to an allergic reaction away from the site of the sting itself. An example would be a sting on someone's arm leading to widespread hives. In some individuals, however, their systemic reaction may progress to anaphylaxis and, while relatively rare, such reactions can be extremely serious.

Fatal insect-venom allergy is seen mainly in adult males, and more than 80 per cent of cases occur in men aged between fifty and sixty years. This difference between the sexes may reflect how commonly men are stung by bees and wasps: men are more likely to be tree-surgeons, builders, roofers, gardeners and to work outdoors, thereby placing them at higher risk of being stung and becoming sensitized. Anaphylaxis to bee stings tends to affect beekeepers and their families, but wasps are not fussy about who they sting, and allergic reactions to wasp stings do not affect one particular group of people. As a wasp does not leave its sting in the victim, it can sting many times. Anaphylaxis to venom often triggers low blood pressure, so patients describe feeling faint and light-headed or dizzy. If this is the case, **under no circumstances** stand up quickly or run away. If you are suffering an anaphylactic reaction and are feeling dizzy and you are still near the wasps or bees and need to get away, then roll or crawl away.

Fortunately there is a potential cure: it is called venom immunotherapy or desensitization. The treatment is offered by allergy clinics and has two stages. The initial phase is called up-dosing, and you receive gradually increasing injections of either bee or wasp venom. Most protocols start at 1/10,000th of a sting and build up to the equivalent of two stings. There are several ways of doing this, and treatment schedules vary between centres and countries. Some protocols involve an intense build-up of injections over a few days, while others involve weekly injections over twelve weeks. This is followed by the second 'maintenance phase'. Lasting three to five years, it involves four to eight weekly top-up injections of venom. At the end of the treatment you will no longer be allergic. If you have suffered a systemic allergic reaction to a bee or wasp sting, then you should be referred to a specialist clinic and this may be a treatment option that is offered to you.

How not to get stung

As a colleague of mine used to say, try not to look or smell like a flower:

- Avoid using strong perfumes during the summer.
- Avoid using strongly scented hairsprays or gels.
- Give brightly coloured clothing or flowery prints a miss.

Food attracts insects, so:

- Avoid eating or drinking outdoors, and spending a long time in locations where food and drinks are being served outdoors.
- Avoid, avoid, avoid rubbish bins, which are a wasp magnet. Likewise, picnic areas or tables with uncleared food outside restaurants.
- Be especially cautious with drinks, as wasps may enter canned drinks or open bottles. Boxed drinks may be safer, but better still is not to drink outdoors.

As for clothing:

- Avoid walking around in bare feet or sandals when outdoors.

2. Speed is of the essence here. **Do not delay** administering adrenaline. Make a note of the time you have given it.
3. If their symptoms are not improving after five minutes, then a second dose can be given.

Step 2: Make sure they stay still.

1. Make sure that the person has stopped moving and is not walking or running around.
2. Standing upright is a feature of fatal anaphylaxis to foods and stings, so make sure that they are not standing. If they feel dizzy, faint or sweaty, then lie them flat. If they are finding it hard to breathe, they may be more comfortable sitting upright.
3. Changes in posture must be very gradual. Suddenly moving from lying flat to sitting up, or from sitting to standing, have been associated with heart attacks and even death.

Step 3: Call an ambulance.

1. Call an ambulance **after** you have administered adrenaline. Explain to the operator that the person is suffering from anaphylaxis. UK readers: do not delay by calling 111 first – go straight to 999.
2. If the person is deteriorating while waiting, call back and check that the ambulance is on its way.
3. If you are in a busy place such as a restaurant or in a hard-to-find location, send someone to direct the ambulance.
4. Even if the person feels better by the time the ambulance arrives, they still need to go to hospital for up to twelve hours' observation, in case the reaction returns.

Step 4: Remember: adrenaline first, everything else afterwards.

1. Antihistamines take thirty to sixty minutes to work.
2. Steroids take at least four hours to work.
3. Antihistamines and steroids can be given, but while they may relieve symptoms such as hives and swelling, they will **not** treat anaphylaxis.

11. Taking the Medicine: The Importance of Drug Allergies

Drug allergy is possibly the most challenging area in allergy because a lot relies on experience, rather than formal guidelines, but for me it is the most rewarding one. My passion for the subject began in the first year of my training, with a perplexing case of anaphylaxis.

Case study: Humphrey

It was a typical morning for Humphrey, a retired banker in his seventies. After his usual breakfast of porridge, a boiled egg with a slice of toast and a cup of tea, he took his usual medications for high blood pressure, high cholesterol and gout. Humphrey then went to read his morning newspaper out in the garden, pausing only to stroke Ulysses, the neighbour's cat.

After finishing his paper he went indoors to get ready for the day. But while he was shaving his face began to swell and he developed a rash. Two minutes later he felt dizzy, clammy and nearly lost consciousness. He was treated for anaphylaxis and was referred by his doctor to the allergy clinic.

By the time Humphrey came to the clinic, he had plucked up the courage to eat the same breakfast again and had drunk countless cups of tea, but suffered no further reaction. He had also taken his same regular tablets. This meant that he had not developed a new allergy to his daily medicines and also eliminated food allergy as the cause (tea drinkers among you will be relieved to hear that allergy to tea is almost unheard of). I skin-tested him for a cat allergy; it was negative. An unsurprising result, because cat allergy triggers asthma and rhinitis, not the hives or low blood pressure that Humphrey experienced.

So, no obvious drug allergy, no food allergy and no cat allergy. I explained to Humphrey that, in exceptionally rare cases, patients can suffer from anaphylaxis with no known cause. I prescribed him an AAI, in case of further reactions, and arranged a follow-up meeting in a few months.

By the time of our next appointment, Humphrey had experienced another episode of anaphylaxis – mercifully stopped in its tracks after he injected adrenaline. We walked through the events, and they were identical to the first episode: breakfast, medication, paper, cat, shaving, anaphylaxis. By now Humphrey was wondering if he was allergic to newspaper ink. He had considered switching to another paper, but decided to continue reading *The Times* wearing gardening gloves. I assured him that his anaphylaxis was not triggered by his newspaper, but he did not look convinced.

Humphrey had a history of anaphylaxis to penicillin, but there was no way he could have mistakenly taken the antibiotic. Searching for answers, on impulse, I handed him my phone and asked him to call his neighbour to find out if Ulysses, the cat, had been taking antibiotics. Ulysses was prone to chest infections, the neighbour explained, requiring several courses of antibiotics in recent months.

For the first and only time in my career, I wrote a letter to a vet about a cat. The vet confirmed that Ulysses had been prescribed a member of the penicillin family of antibiotics called co-amoxiclav at the time of both of Humphrey's anaphylactic reactions.

Humphrey was therefore invited for drug allergy testing and had a positive skin-prick test to penicillin. I had diluted the solution a thousand-fold – a single drop of solution, made up of 999 parts water and one part penicillin, was enough to produce an itchy bump where I scratched his skin. I concluded that trace quantities of penicillin excreted in Ulysses's urine, skin and saliva had caused both of Humphrey's anaphylactic reactions.

Now Humphrey was an extreme case: I have only a handful of patients with such a severe drug allergy. Even individuals with life-threatening drug allergy usually react only when they themselves take the drug. However, his story does underline that drug allergy is a very real problem and can be extremely serious – drug allergy is the leading cause of fatal anaphylaxis in Australia, New Zealand, the UK, Brazil and the USA.[1] Up to 20 per cent of drug-related anaphylaxis deaths in Europe, and up to 75 per cent in the US, are caused by penicillin.[2]

However, another critical issue is the mislabelling of some-one as allergic to a drug when they are in fact suffering from a side-effect or symptoms of illness or infection. One study esti-mated that, in England alone, just under three million people have an incorrect label of being allergic to penicillin.[3] And an incorrect label can be as serious as a drug allergy in itself, because it can bar a patient from a potentially lifesaving group of medicines.

The bottom line is: drug allergy is important, and there-fore getting an accurate diagnosis is even more important. People come into my clinic believing they are allergic to a drug and having carried that label for decades, but within a few short hours we often find out this isn't the case. 'De-labelling' can be incredibly satisfying for both doctor and patient and has the potential to be life-changing in a positive way. And the good news is that these tests, when undertaken by a trained professional, will bring clarity. They will almost always confirm whether you are a member of the drug-allergy club so that alternative medications can be discussed, or will confidently rule out drug allergy once and for all.

In this chapter I will delve into exactly what drug allergy is. I'll take you through the discussions and tests that you can expect to have if you are referred to a specialist allergy clinic. The key groups of drugs that I'll be looking at are:

- Antibiotics, such as penicillin
- Painkillers
- Local anaesthetic
- General anaesthetic.

The pitfalls of an incorrect drug-allergy label

Most people who believe they are allergic to medication are not – particularly when it comes to antibiotics.

Let me give you an example: about 10 per cent of the UK population are recorded by their family doctor as being allergic to penicillin and have often acquired this label after developing a rash, while taking penicillin in childhood or adulthood. It is thought that more than 90 per cent of these labels are incorrect.[4] Penicillin is an A-lister among antibiotics. It is widely used to treat skin infections, chest infections and urinary-tract infections. Patients who are recorded as being allergic to penicillin are prescribed alternative antibiotics, which may be less effective or leave them vulnerable to infections with multidrug-resistant bacteria or superbugs.

It is entirely natural to be concerned if you develop a rash while on antibiotics, but in the vast majority of cases the rash is actually triggered by the infecting virus or bacteria rather than by the drug treatment. The difficulty is that there is no way to be certain, without drug-allergy investigation in a specialist clinic. And so doctors are forced to err on the side of caution and record a patient as being penicillin-allergic – a label that usually remains unchallenged throughout their life. That is why, as well as confirming an allergy, removing the label of drug allergy forms a big part of what allergy clinics do.

So if you have a label of drug allergy that you suspect is inaccurate, talk to your doctor and ask to be referred to a specialist clinic to get a firm answer. Whatever you do, **do not** be tempted to take matters into your hands and try medication to which you are recorded as allergic.

Myth-busting: there are lots of them!

'But I've taken drug X plenty of times before, so I can't possibly be allergic'

This is something I frequently hear from patients in my drug-allergy clinic. This is not the case, or nobody would develop any new drug allergies. Unfortunately you can develop a drug allergy at any point, so having tolerated a drug previously does not mean you won't develop an allergy to it in the future. The likelihood of becoming allergic to many drugs, particularly antibiotics, increases with the number of times you are exposed to them and how it is administered (if it is rubbed into the skin or injected into a vein or muscle, developing an allergy is more likely[5]). Therefore drug allergy usually develops in adulthood . . .

'One dose is all it takes'

Drug allergy does not usually 'build up' to some sort of crescendo over a period of time. If you are allergic, then a single dose of a drug will be enough to tip you into an immediate allergic reaction.

'Mixing drug X and drug Y has made me allergic'

Again this is something I hear on a regular basis, but an allergic reaction will not be caused by several drugs combining in your stomach.

'I am allergic to shellfish – I need to avoid iodine'

If you are allergic to shellfish you do not need to avoid drugs containing iodine, such as iodine-based antiseptics or iodine-containing contrast media (chemical substances that are injected into the body to enhance X-rays, so that it is easier for specialists to spot abnormalities). Shellfish allergy is due to a specific IgE to certain proteins in the shellfish, and not to iodine, and there is no need for concern.

'I am allergic to hen's egg, so what about the MMR vaccine?'

If you have a history of anaphylaxis to hen's eggs, you can still receive the measles, mumps and rubella (MMR) vaccine with no special precautions. The MMR vaccine is grown on cells called fibroblasts that are derived from chick embryos and therefore do not contain hen's-egg protein (or if they do contain traces of protein, the levels are too low to cause an allergic reaction).

'I am allergic to hen's egg, so what about the flu vaccine?'

People with egg allergy do not need to avoid the influenza vaccine, and this includes both adults and children with a history of anaphylaxis to egg. In the UK the only exception is adults and children who have had anaphylaxis to egg that is so severe they have required intensive-care admission. Influenza vaccines are derived from the influenza virus, which is grown in hen's egg but, once purified, the amount of residual egg protein remaining is 2,000–5,000-fold lower than the amount that is likely to trigger reactions in people with an egg allergy. Guidance and influenza vaccines vary between countries, but in the UK the Green Book gives specific information to family doctors about which influenza vaccines they can or cannot administer to their patients (see Further Reading and Resources on page 221).

Tests for drug allergy

There are four stages in the investigation and diagnosis of drug allergy (see the text below and the illustration opposite). Drug-allergy blood tests are available, but they are rarely reliable enough to make or exclude a diagnosis of drug allergy.

Not every patient will need to complete every step: for example, patients with very low-risk drug-allergy history can go direct to a drug challenge without skin-testing. But if you do have to complete each stage, the clarity of finding out whether you are truly allergic to a medication or not will be worth it.

Step 1: History

This is essentially a discussion of what happened, including:

- **How soon after taking the medicine did a reaction occur?** Immediate reactions to drugs are usually within the hour and often within minutes, although reactions to NSAIDS can take up to two hours, to allow for the coating surrounding the drug to dissolve. If antibiotic allergy is suspected, knowing where in the course the reaction occurs is critical. Due to the mechanisms involved

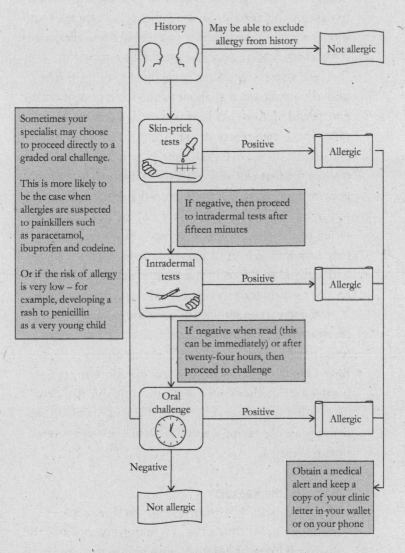

History — May be able to exclude allergy from history → Not allergic

Sometimes your specialist may choose to proceed directly to a graded oral challenge.

This is more likely to be the case when allergies are suspected to painkillers such as paracetamol, ibuprofen and codeine.

Or if the risk of allergy is very low – for example, developing a rash to penicillin as a very young child

Skin-prick tests — Positive → Allergic

If negative, then proceed to intradermal tests after fifteen minutes

Intradermal tests — Positive → Allergic

If negative when read (this can be immediately) or after twenty-four hours, then proceed to challenge

Oral challenge — Positive → Allergic

Negative

Not allergic

Obtain a medical alert and keep a copy of your clinic letter in your wallet or on your phone

Investigating drug allergy

in immediate allergic reactions, it is virtually impossible to develop this reaction midway through a course of anti-biotics as it would mean that you had become allergic over a few hours, which would be incredibly rare.

- **Delayed reactions**: Allergic reactions to drugs can be delayed, usually starting about twenty-four hours into the course and up to weeks later (although the latter is very rare). Immediate reactions are, however, far more common and are the focus of this chapter. A rash (not hives) is frequently the first clue that something is amiss. More usually patients report flat, red patches on the skin, which merge to form a rash. Other symptoms may include a fever, blistering of the skin, mouth or genitals. Severe reactions may even lead to liver or kidney damage. Drugs associated with delayed reactions include anti-epileptic medications, certain medicines to treat gout, iodine contrast media for X-rays, and certain families of antibiotics. Delayed drug reactions are a specialist field in themselves, and much more detail is beyond the scope of this book.
- **Side-effects**: Your doctor may ask questions to try to distinguish whether your symptoms were due to a drug allergy or due to drug side-effects. Nausea, vomiting and diarrhoea while taking a medication are side-effects and not an allergy.

Keep the packaging

If you suspect that your reaction is due to a medication, jot down the active ingredients and the dose and bring the details with you to the allergy clinic. Alternatively, take a photograph of the packaging. This is especially the case with branded medicines. For example, Anadin is a UK painkiller brand with a range of preparations: Anadin Extra contains both aspirin and paracetamol; Anadin Ultra contains ibuprofen; and original Anadin contains aspirin only.

Step 2: Skin-prick testing

Skin-prick testing involves placing small drops of the drug that you suspect you may be allergic to on your forearm (or sometimes your back) and pricking the skin, using a sterile lancet. This allows a small amount of the drug to enter the skin. If you are allergic, you may develop a small itchy bump, called a wheal, at the site of the test. Often this is surrounded by a red flare. A positive test occurs within fifteen minutes of testing.

Step 3: Intradermal testing

If skin-prick tests are negative, the next stage is intradermal testing, a far more sensitive test. Using a small and very thin needle, a diluted amount of the drug is injected just below the skin surface to raise a very small bump. If an intradermal test is positive, the bump grows by at least 3mm and will not flatten. It may also become itchy and red.

Skin-prick and intradermal testing are useful when investigating patients with a suspected allergy to penicillin, local and general anaesthetic agents and antiseptic agents such as chlorhexidine. However, these tests are rarely of any use when investigating allergy to painkillers such as ibuprofen, paracetamol or codeine. Nor are they helpful in the diagnosis of allergy to certain antibiotics such as clarithromycin, trimethoprim or nitrofurantoin. This is probably because reactions to these antibiotics are non-IgE-mediated.

Step 4: Graded drug challenge

This involves trying a drug again in increasing amounts, to confirm that you are not allergic. Drug challenge is routinely carried out following a negative skin-prick and intradermal tests to certain drugs such as penicillin and local anaesthetics to confirm that you are not allergic. Patients may also go directly to a drug challenge to eliminate allergy to drugs, where skin testing is not useful. Drug-challenge testing takes several hours, and sometimes patients are asked to continue taking the drug at home for a further few days.

Please be reassured that drug-allergy investigations – be it skin-prick or intradermal tests, or drug challenge – are extremely safe when undertaken by an experienced specialist. I have successfully challenged several thousand patients to a wide range of medications and have never had to admit a patient as a result of an allergic reaction. There is no safer environment to do this than in a clinic, with an experienced team and all the equipment and drugs on hand to treat an allergic reaction, such as in a large centre like ours.

Different drug allergies explained
Penicillin allergy

Every morning when I go to my clinic I walk past a plaque commemorating Nobel Prize-winner Sir Alexander Fleming, who discovered penicillin while working at St Mary's. According to my mentor Bill Frankland, he did not much like the idea that allergy to penicillin was going to become an increasing problem. Initially there was just one penicillin, but now the word refers to a group of antibiotics that includes amoxicillin, ampicillin, co-amoxiclav, benzylpenicillin and flucloxacillin – think of the name 'penicillin' like a family surname. For a long time a label of penicillin allergy, even if inaccurate in the vast majority of patients, was not seen as particularly worrisome.

This changed in 2014 when a large study by the American allergist Eric Macy found that people with a label of penicillin allergy were significantly more vulnerable to infection from superbugs, such as MRSA.[6] They were also at higher risk of developing a contagious, aggressive diarrhoea with a bacterium called *Clostridium difficile*. Macy's work represented a watershed moment for drug allergy. From thereon in, numerous papers have been published demonstrating that a label of penicillin allergy is associated with worse health outcomes. In 2019 a huge UK study involving data from two million patients found that the label of 'penicillin allergy' was associated with a 1.3-fold risk of treatment failure.[7] And in July 2021 the impact of a label of penicillin allergy was evaluated in more than 26,000 COVID-19-positive patients. The authors found the label was associated with a higher risk of hospitalization, intensive-care admission and the need for life-support. This was surprising, as COVID-19 is a viral infection and therefore antibiotics are not useful; but one tentative explanation is that COVID-19 infection can make patients more vulnerable to bacterial pneumonia and, if penicillin is off-limits, then a bacterial pneumonia is harder to treat.[8]

So if your medical records note that you are 'allergic to penicillin', talk to your family doctor to try to find out why this label has been applied and which penicillin is thought to have caused the reaction.

If you are having to: i) avoid multiple groups of antibiotics because of suspected drug allergy, or ii) are vulnerable to infections because you are not able to take penicillin, approach your family doctor and find out about access to drug-allergy testing locally. Access to services may be patchy, but ask for a referral.

Allergy to painkillers (analgesics)

About one in five patients referred to my drug-allergy clinic are thought to be allergic to painkillers. These drugs fall into three main groups:

1. NSAIDS such as ibuprofen, aspirin and diclofenac
2. Paracetamol
3. Opiates such as morphine, pethidine, tramadol, codeine and fentanyl.

NSAIDs: This group is responsible for the majority of painkiller-related allergic reactions, and sometimes these reactions can occur up to two hours after taking the painkiller, due to the tablets being enterically coated.

NSAIDs are also associated with a particular type of asthma called aspirin-exacerbated respiratory disease. This condition starts in adulthood, and patients develop nasal polyps, asthma and rhinosinusitis. Taking an NSAID in this group of asthmatics can trigger life-threatening asthma.

In individuals with non-allergic urticaria or non-allergic hives, NSAIDS may trigger or worsen an outbreak and should be avoided (see Chapter 12 for more information).

NSAIDS can also cause certain allergic reactions to foods, such as in wheat-dependent exercise-induced anaphylaxis and allergy to lipid transfer proteins (see Chapter 7).

If you think you are allergic to one NSAID, you should avoid the entire group until you have seen a specialist.

Paracetamol: This is one of the most commonly used analgesics and has an excellent safety record when used in the right doses. Paracetamol allergy is rare – and more than 95 per cent of people with an allergy to NSAIDs will be able to take paracetamol safely[9] – but it does exist. At my clinic we are increasingly seeing patients of any age who are developing allergic reactions to paracetamol, but for the most part the reactions are mainly those of hives and swelling, rather than anaphylaxis.

Opiates: These are stronger painkillers and allergy to them is incredibly rare; I have never seen a single case in my career. However, intensely itchy skin is a common side-effect of opiates, and this can sometimes be confused with allergy. Opiates are usually part of an epidural, and many anaesthetists will warn their patients to expect itchy skin.

> **Read the box**
> **If you think you are allergic to painkillers, read the labels carefully: paracetamol and NSAIDS are commonly found in medications for headache, period pain and sinus pain, and in cold and flu tablets and muscle rubs (these often contain**

low doses of diclofenac, ibuprofen or aspirin-derivatives – salicylic acid and salicylates – but nonetheless may contain enough drug to trigger an allergic reaction). Better still, buy from a pharmacy rather than a supermarket shelf, so that you can get advice from a pharmacist.

Allergy to local anaesthetic

I see dozens of patients every year who are referred to me to investigate a suspected allergy to local anaesthetic, but when we skin-test and challenge these patients, they are almost never allergic. So what is going on? Many patients are referred following a visit to the dentist or after a coil insertion, and have become unwell shortly after local anaesthetic was administered. However, one of the following problems can often be mistaken for an allergic reaction:

- Local anaesthetic administered at the dentist's is usually combined with adrenaline, to reduce bleeding into the mouth during surgery. When too much adrenaline is absorbed into the circulation, it can trigger a rapid pulse, raised blood pressure, tremor and a feeling of restlessness.
- Fainting can also mimic an allergic reaction. Symptoms prior to passing out can include sweating, feeling light-headed, feeling sick and passing out. Stimulating the neck of the womb during coil insertion (when local anaesthetic is often used) is well described to cause this.
- Anxiety can result in a racing heart, feeling faint and nausea.

This is another drug-allergy label that, if incorrect, can have implications on your healthcare in the future. It's better to get a referral to a drug-allergy clinic for further investigation, otherwise you potentially face having to avoid local anaesthetic for the rest of your life.

If allergy is suspected, ask your dentist to write to your family doctor, documenting the drugs you were given, the amount of each drug and the reaction you had (don't forget to ask for a copy, too). Your family doctor should then refer you to a specialist allergy clinic for investigation.

Anaphylactic reactions during surgery (perioperative anaphylaxis): the drug-allergy detectives

Nearly three million general anaesthetics are given to patients in the UK every year and allergic reactions during surgery are fortunately rare (about 1 in 10,000 patients in the UK). However, the implications of a reaction are considerable and, if the cause is not discovered, it makes further surgery a hazardous undertaking. However, identifying which drug triggered a reaction isn't always easy. That is because multiple drugs are given during an anaesthetic – the average is eight, but sometimes it's many more.

So those patients referred to an allergy clinic with a suspected allergic reaction to general anaesthetic challenge specialists, like myself, to turn into detectives to get to the root cause. The patient was asleep, so there is no history to be had, and we therefore ask the anaesthetist to send us information about what happened at the time, or from the 'crime scene'.

In 2018 the UK's Royal College of Anaesthetists published the largest-ever study of its kind into life-threatening anaphylaxis during surgery.[10] I was one of the expert authors in this study and we analysed data from every case in UK hospitals over a twelve-month period. Antibiotics accounted for 47 per cent of perioperative anaphylactic reactions, followed by muscle relaxants (33 per cent), the antiseptic chlorhexidine (9 per cent) and patent blue dye (5 per cent), which is a dye used during certain breast surgeries. So anaesthetic agents themselves (the drugs that send you to sleep) almost never caused an allergic reaction in themselves.

If you have had a suspected serious allergic reaction during surgery it should be investigated without delay. On discharge from hospital, you should be provided with a letter from your anaesthetist detailing what happened and which drugs you received. Your family doctor should then refer you to a specialist allergy clinic.

If you think you had a previous perioperative anaphylactic reaction, but it was not investigated, ask your family doctor to contact the hospital and try and find out what happened. If doubts remain about whether or not you are allergic, then your doctor should refer you to an allergy clinic, which will try and help. And if you are due to have surgery soon, it is **essential** that you inform staff you may have had an allergic reaction before.

12. Red Herrings: When you Think you are Allergic . . . But You Aren't

I had been qualified as a doctor for three years, working long hours and nervously waiting for my professional exam results. Without obtaining my MRCP (Membership of the Royal College of Physicians), I wouldn't be able to progress on to specialist training. I was feeling the pressure. To cap it all, I had a bad episode of sinusitis. My family doctor had prescribed me penicillin, but I still felt rough. I woke up in the early hours and took a couple of ibuprofen. I then hauled myself into work. On my hour-long commute other passengers were giving me strange looks. This was unusual for a packed London Tube train in rush hour, where the unwritten rule is to avoid eye contact, but I felt too ill to think much of it. I felt hot and put it down to a fever. My face felt full and tight, and I thought this was due to my sinuses.

It was only when I walked onto the ward and saw myself in a mirror that I realized that my face was swollen. My neck and arms were also covered in large, itchy hives or, to give them their medical term, urticaria. My consultant took one look at me, likened my appearance to Shrek and sent me home, proclaiming that I would 'frighten' his patients.

On the way out he stated that I was clearly allergic to penicillin and that I would be a good teaching case for the medical students. It was only several years later that I realized he was completely wrong. I hadn't suffered an allergic reaction at all.

Let me tell you about the biggest red herring of them all: non-allergic urticaria and angioedema.

Urticaria and angioedema

About one in five of us will develop an outbreak of urticaria at some point, yet despite this, it is rarely taught about in medical school. And these red, raised itchy wheals cause a lot of stress, because frequently both doctors and patients assume they must be due to an allergy. So much so that a study of allergy-clinic referrals in Ireland found that 71 per cent of referrals for allergy investigation requested food-allergy testing, although chronic urticaria actually accounted for more than half of these cases.[1]

The wheals that characterize urticaria usually disappear within minutes to hours, but can come and go for days or weeks at a time. If the welts appear on most days for more than six weeks, it is termed chronic urticaria.[2]

Angioedema is part of the same spectrum, but describes deeper swellings in the skin – most frequently around the eyes, lips, face and occasionally the tongue or soft palate. It isn't usually itchy, but the skin can feel tight and uncomfortable. And although alarming, it is usually not life-threatening, unless it is caused by a group of drugs used to treat high blood pressure called ACE inhibitors (ACE-I) or is due to a rare enzyme deficiency called C1 esterase inhibitor deficiency.

So if it is not an allergy, what causes urticaria and angioedema?

You may remember mast cells from back in Chapter 1. Sometimes the mast cells that live in your skin can become 'hyperactive' and release their histamine. This mischief can lead to urticaria and/or angioedema, and it may be mild and a one-off or it may cause misery and lead to chronic symptoms. It is not connected to allergy. Specialists can usually tell if your urticaria or angioedema is due to an allergy, by examining the circumstances leading up to it and its duration.

Are your urticaria and angiodema due to a food allergy?

	Unlikely food allergy	Likely food allergy
Timing	Outbreaks are random and do not relate clearly to eating certain foods.	Usually occurs within minutes to an hour of eating a suspect food, and very rarely up to two hours later. If you don't eat the suspect food, then you are well.
Allergen exposure	No clear allergen exposure. If you go to sleep without hives and wake up with hives, allergy is almost never the cause.	Urticaria and/or angioedema occurs soon after eating a common food allergen, such as egg, peanut or shellfish.
Duration	Lasts from days to weeks.	Resolves within twenty-four hours.
Other symptoms	None. Just urticaria and/or angioedema.	Itching of mouth/hard palate. Difficulty breathing. Feeling light-headed or faint. Persistent coughing.
Recurrence	Randomly. If you are experiencing chronic hives that wax and wane, allergy is rarely the cause.	Only when exposed to the suspect allergen; if the allergen is avoided, then the symptoms resolve.

Prognosis	It usually burns out over time.	If it develops in adulthood, food allergy usually persists.
Patient	Can occur at any age and affects both atopic and non-atopic individuals.	Usually seen in younger patients, who may have a history of eczema, asthma and rhinitis. It is very unusual to develop a new food allergy in your fifties, sixties or beyond.

One of the most frustrating things for patients – quite aside from the rash or swelling itself – is its significant impact on their quality of life, work, sleep and relationships. The absence of a clear trigger adds to the frustration. 'If only I knew what was causing it' is a lament I frequently hear. However, looking beyond allergy as a cause may reveal a trigger – you just need to think in a different way.

Triggers of non-allergic urticaria and angioedema

- **Bacterial or viral infection** is probably one of the most common triggers.
- **Stress** is also well recognized to precipitate episodes. In my experience, this can be either sudden episodes of stress (I recall a patient telling me that she broke out into hives when she was clubbing and her handbag was stolen) or chronic stress, caused by traumatic life events such as bereavement or divorce.[3]
- **NSAIDS** can aggravate urticaria and angioedema, so they should be avoided where possible. However, low-dose 'junior' aspirin (75 mg) does not usually worsen it, so if

you are taking a low dose aspirin to thin your blood, do not suddenly stop it.

- **Physical triggers** cause hives in some people, including cold (such as cold air, water or ice), a change in temperature, heat or even sunlight (solar).
- **Dermatographism** is another variation of urticaria, which literally means 'skin writing'. This occurs when a patient's skin is lightly scratched or rubbed and, within minutes, raised welts appear along the lines of the scratch.
- **Delayed pressure urticaria**, where swellings can be painful – such as after carrying heavy bags or wearing high heels – is rare, but can be debilitating.
- **Cholinergic urticaria** is where a rise in core body temperature causes hives to emerge, for example, after exercise (sweating), spicy food or with a fever.

Treatment

The mainstay of treatment is antihistamines.

1. If your urticaria is occurring several times a week or more, a daily dose of a long-acting non-sedating antihistamine, such as cetirizine or loratadine, is the best place to start. If this does not help, talk to your family doctor, because up to four tablets a day may be needed. Antihistamines sold over the counter will give the dose needed to treat nose and eye symptoms, but the skin is a huge organ and more antihistamine may be needed, so don't be alarmed by the number of tablets you may be asked to take. If antihistamines do not completely control symptoms, an asthma medication called montelukast may

be added. This blocks the effects of a chemical released from mast cells called leukotrienes.

2. Menthol in aqueous cream can also be useful, because it cools as it evaporates from your skin and can help with itchiness.

3. Your doctor may prescribe oral steroids to settle angioedema, but these will not help urticaria.

In a minority of patients, treatments started by a specialist clinic may be required.

ACE-inhibitor-induced angioedema

If you are referred to an allergy clinic with a history of angioedema, the first thing the allergist will usually do is scan your list of medications and check if you are taking an ACE-I. These medications are brilliantly effective at lowering blood pressure and are widely used. They usually end in -*pril* – examples include benazepril, enalapril, lisinopril, perindopril and ramipril. If you are taking an ACE-I, then your allergist will likely call or write to you (and your family doctor) and advise you to immediately stop the ACE-I. This is because angioedema triggered by ACE-I can, on rare occasions, involve the throat and be very serious. More frequently, however, it involves the face, lips, gums and tongue. Swelling of just one side of the tongue is typical. A big diagnostic clue is that urticaria is **not** a feature.

The diagnosis of ACE-I angioedema is made on history alone. For a medication that is so frequently prescribed, few doctors are aware of this side-effect and it is not emphasized in medical training. Yet it is estimated that ACE-I angioedema affects up to 0.6 per cent of people taking the medication.[4]

People can take ACE-I for months and even years and then suddenly, seemingly out of nowhere, the swelling begins.[5] Asian and Afro-Caribbean patients are more vulnerable. More confusion arises because, after the initial episode of swelling, there may be no further swelling for months, despite taking the medication every day; and then, suddenly, it recurs. I wish we knew why, but nobody is really sure.

Unfortunately there is no 'test' to confirm ACE-I angi-oedema: it is what is known as a clinical diagnosis, so it is made on medical history alone. Therefore if you don't sus-pect it, you will miss it. Thankfully, discontinuing the ACE-I will resolve the swelling, although it may take several months to settle completely and there may be episodes of recurrence in between.

13. What to Do If You Think You Have an Allergy

We've now covered the key triggers, symptoms, treatments and coping strategies for everything from rhinitis to food allergy. Maybe you already have a confirmed diagnosis and are on a treatment plan. Or perhaps you have had a suspicion for some time that you might be allergic and now want to do something about it.

This chapter is about taking you through those all-important medical consultations. From preparing for your appointment, to what you can expect when you visit an allergy clinic, it will help you get the most out of your appointments.

Family doctor: your first port of call

If you have health insurance, then in many countries you can contact a specialist and book an appointment directly. However, if you live in a country with nationalized healthcare (or your health insurance requires it), your journey to see us will start with a visit to your family doctor, who will then refer you to a specialist clinic.

Appointments may be short – the average family doctor's appointment is 9.2 minutes in the UK – but with some preparation and careful questions, you should be able to have a satisfying consultation. Write down what bothers you the most, and what you want to achieve in the appointment. Save these notes on your phone to use as a prompt. If you have a lot to discuss, request a double appointment. Before your consultation:

1. Make a list of your symptoms.
2. Note the timing, particularly for suspected food allergy: how soon after being exposed to the suspected allergen did your symptoms start?
3. For rhinitis or asthma, note down any treatments you have tried and whether or not they have helped.
4. Take a photo of any rashes, to show your doctor.

At the appointment explain how your symptoms are impacting your quality of life, so that your doctor understands what life is like in your shoes. For example, 'I have terrible hay fever, my eyes itch and burn, and my nose is running. I have tried antihistamine X and nose spray Y, and I still am no better. I am using two packs of tissues a day. I cannot go out with the kids, I cannot sleep and I am worried about driving because I am sneezing so much. Please can you refer me to see a specialist.'

Remember that if you have had a significant reaction to a food or a venom, you don't need to wait until you go to an allergy clinic to be prescribed an autoinjector.

How long will it take for my referral to come through?

This varies hugely between clinics and countries. In the UK and some other countries, redeployment of allergy-clinic staff during the COVID-19 pandemic and social distancing have led to a substantial increase in waiting times in NHS clinics (several months). With the uptake of vaccinations, we are hopeful that things will return to normal, although the backlog of patients may take a while to clear. Regardless of the waiting time, it is good to keep notes of what happened when you reacted, because it can be hard to remember, even weeks later. If for some reason you can't make your appointment, call as soon as possible to rearrange it, and that slot can then be offered to someone else.

What to expect when you visit an allergy clinic

I am hugely proud to work at the UK's oldest allergy clinic alongside a fantastic team of specialist doctors, nurses and dieticians, who are passionate about improving people's health and well-being. Behind-the-scenes managers, administrative and secretarial staff are all contributing to a smooth-running service. Thousands of patients come through our doors every single year, and no two cases of allergy are ever the same, but here is some advice on what you should expect when you come to an allergy clinic like mine.

History-taking

When you see an allergist, expect far more in-depth history-taking than with your family doctor, especially during the first visit. At this initial consultation I spend a lot of time trying to understand my patient's story, and this is the most important part of that appointment. Allergy is primarily diagnosed on history, and since our patients often have eczema, rhinitis, asthma and food allergy there is a lot to cover, and consultations are often fairly lengthy. We will drill down into the detail, particularly if a food allergy is suspected.

If you think you have reacted to a food, we may ask for an ingredient list (if we don't know the ingredients in what you ate, it makes investigating it much harder). If you have a history of rhinitis or urticaria, we will ask you about the names of medicines that you have tried and which have helped or not helped you. We don't want to suggest something that already hasn't worked.

Many aspects of allergies may change over time, especially in younger patients, so our approach to treatment is not 'set and forget', but we will revisit how they are doing over time. Some patients may be asked to return to a specialist clinic, such as our drug-allergy clinic, a food-challenge clinic or for immunotherapy.

Consultations during COVID

Since the onset of COVID-19, many hospitals have tried to reduce footfall, because nobody wants their patients to catch COVID by attending an appointment. So your initial consultation may be via telephone or video-link, and then you will be invited to the clinic for skin-prick testing or a food or drug challenge. Insurance companies are also now more open to online or phone consultations, known as telemedicine consultations. Your specialist will be more than aware that managing allergies during the pandemic has been tricky, but allergists have an ability to ask very detailed questions and come up with a plan, so a lot can be achieved even remotely. One size doesn't fit all, but in my experience most people like the convenience of tele-medicine, so it could be here to stay, at least for some groups of patients. For more about navigating a tele-medicine appointment, see Appendix 2 (page 202).

Do I need to bring anything with me?

Your clinic should write to you with specific instructions on what to bring, but if you think you may be allergic to fruit, vegetables or shellfish, you will often be asked to bring a small sample with you for skin-prick testing. The same applies to unusual foods. It is important to keep foods for skin-prick testing packed separately to avoid cross-contamination – for example, bring in a whole apple and whole grapes, rather than mixed together in a fruit salad. If you have a suspected drug allergy, bring with you the medication you think you reacted to or take photos of the packaging, including the name and ingredients list, and keep it on your phone.

What tests might I undergo?

Testing is very much guided by your history. Depending on your suspected allergen, you may have one or more of the following tests:

- **Skin-prick test**: This involves placing small drops of liquid (many pharmaceutical companies make these) containing an allergen onto your forearm (in very young children or if you have severe eczema, your back may be used) and pricking the skin using a sterile lancet. If you're allergic to the substance, an itchy, red bump will appear within fifteen minutes.

- **Skin-prick test to fresh foods**: This is the same as a skin-prick test, but involves pricking the skin with a fresh food substance rather than a standardized skin-prick test solution. It allows very accurate skin-prick testing – for example, to peach skin and peach flesh.

  <u>Top tip</u>
  Wear comfortable clothing that allows easy access to your forearm for skin-prick testing.

  - **Specific IgE test: A blood test to measure different IgE antibodies against allergens may be checked – for example, to pollens or foods. Sometimes component allergen tests will be requested, which enable your allergist to identify exactly which protein in the food you may be reacting to.**
  - **Food challenge: This is where increasing amounts of a particular food are fed to a person while under medical supervision. It is generally used by allergy specialists to help determine whether or not a food allergy exists.**
  - **Drug challenge: This is where a person is given increasing amounts of a particular drug under allergist supervision. It is commonly used to confirm or eliminate a diagnosis of drug allergy (see Chapter 11).**

How long will I be at the clinic?

Skin-prick tests and specific IgE blood tests are not a diagnosis, rather they support a diagnosis. Therefore the format of first appointments tends to be history-taking → skin-prick tests → discuss results. So each first appointment is like two consultations in one, and you should keep at least two hours free. Follow-up appointments may be shorter.

Drug-allergy testing can last several hours, and a food challenge around half a day. Try and clear your diary after the appointment, so that you don't feel hassled. Bring a magazine, listen to a podcast and try and relax – and bring your phone charger (most clinics won't have a spare one for you to use!).

I'm taking antihistamines – should I stop taking them ahead of my appointment?

You will often be asked to stop taking antihistamines a few days before your appointment, as they may interfere with skin-prick tests. Follow the advice of the clinic and, if in doubt, call to check.

Make sure you leave the consultation feeling clear about what will happen next: will you need more testing and, if so, when? Are there any strategies you should be adopting? What is the treatment plan?

14. Turning Off the Tap: Eczema and Allergy Prevention

By the time you are an adult, allergies are usually set in stone, but in children's allergy there are intensive efforts to try and stop them from developing in the first place and to halt their progression.

Case study: Rhiannon

Rhiannon, now nineteen, is one of my many patients with the full burden of allergic disease. She first developed eczema in infancy, allergies to hen's egg and peanut by the time she was six months, and asthma and rhinitis in later childhood. She was teased at school about her appearance – her eczema caused her skin to dry, flake and crust, making her self-conscious. Her skin would bleed if she scratched it too much. Her sleep was poor. She would often return home from school in tears, and her mother told me that she felt powerless to help her daughter. Getting ready for school took hours, due to lengthy skincare routines, and Rhiannon would frequently run into trouble with her teachers for being late. She was eventually referred to a specialist allergy clinic, where she learned about skincare routines, and her food allergy, eczema, asthma and rhinitis were all managed. As she grew older, her need for medication diminished and her eczema naturally improved, although her skin remains dry and she will probably need to moisturize regularly for the rest of her life. Rhiannon also outgrew her allergy to egg. With knowledge and specialist support, her ability to explain her allergies to others improved and her confidence grew. Rhiannon is now studying medicine and told me that her decision to train to be a doctor was directly influenced by her experiences as she was growing up.

Rhiannon's journey of developing different allergies (starting with eczema, progressing to food allergy, with the later emergence of asthma and rhinitis) is what allergy specialists call 'the atopic march' – and it is our mission to halt it. In the last twenty years we have made considerable progress in learning what we should *and* shouldn't do to prevent allergy. Here I want to share with you the latest developments.

In this chapter we will look at eczema and its relationship with food allergy, before moving on to eczema treatment and allergy prevention. There are also plenty of helpful hints and coping strategies along the way.

Eczema and food allergy: separating fact from fiction

'Food allergy doesn't cause eczema, eczema causes food allergy,' according to the US allergist Dr Brian Schroer.

Yet one of the biggest myths is that this common condition is due to a 'hidden' food allergy. In fact eczema is largely genetic and this is why it often runs in families. The problem is a weak skin barrier that leaks moisture. Food allergy can be a complication of eczema, but it is not the cause of the dry, itchy and inflamed skin that causes so much heartache. In a bid to 'solve' eczema, patients request (and doctors often agree to) a test for a food allergy, but false-positive blood tests in eczema are extremely common. When a positive test returns, it is tempting to start eliminating foods from the diet, in the hope that this eases symptoms. Yet cutting out foods that are being eaten, without signs of allergy, can be problematic for two reasons:

- Removing a food from the diet, such as eggs, may predispose someone (especially if they have eczema) to actually **develop** a life-threatening food allergy because the immune system 'forgets' it is safe. This is especially true in young children, but we see it in adults, too. With the widespread popularity of veganism, it is unclear whether this will translate into adults developing new egg and dairy allergies in the future. However since most food allergies develop in early childhood, I remain optimistic that this won't be the case.

- Once a food is eliminated for several weeks in a young child with eczema, the only way to safely reintroduce it is with specialist help. Often a food challenge (see page 109) in a hospital setting is required, and access to such investigations can be limited. If multiple foods are eliminated, it can therefore take years to find out if someone is allergic or not.

The real relationship between eczema and food allergy

Eczema in infancy is the single biggest risk factor for developing a food allergy. The earlier the eczema starts and the more severe it is, the greater the risk of food allergy.

For example, an infant who develops severe eczema (requiring prescription steroid creams) between birth and three months of age has a 50 per cent chance of developing a food allergy. The risk drops to 10 per cent in an infant who develops eczema aged ten to twelve months and who only requires daily moisturization. The risk of a child with no eczema developing a food allergy sits at around 3 per cent.[1]

Ultimately it's your genes that hold the casting vote as to whether or not you develop eczema. Imagine your skin like a brick wall, and the cement that holds the bricks together is crumbling – that's what is happening in eczema. There are mutations in the gene that produce the cement (a protein called filaggrin). Without enough filaggrin to build a strong skin barrier, bacteria, viruses and food allergens can easily enter your skin, while moisture can easily escape. Once food allergens and microbes start to penetrate the skin, your immune system thinks it is under attack and may start treating foods as allergens. This triggers an inflammatory immune response, hence the angry red skin that is often seen in eczema. In addition eczema is prone to becoming infected with the bacteria *Staphylococcus aureus*, which forms a biofilm across the skin. This pathogen in particular interacts with the immune system to promote allergic responses.[2]

How to tell if your child has eczema – and how you can treat it

In infants, eczema will often start with dry, rough skin on the face and scalp that spreads. Typically the cheeks are involved, but the nose is spared. In Caucasian children eczema is most likely to affect the skin creases, neck, back of the knees and inside of the elbows and will often be red in appearance. Patches of eczema in children from Asian or Afro-Caribbean families may also be present on the front of the knees and back of the elbows, and might appear purplish, brownish or greyish. A great resource to help guide you is Skin Deep, a free online library of images showing medical conditions, including eczema, in a range of skin tones.[3] And as a heads up, young babies may not be able to reach where they are itching, so you may notice them wriggling on the mattress if their back or scalp is itching and rubbing their feet on their shins because they cannot grab them and give them a good scratch.

How to treat eczema in children

Regular skincare is essential to prevent flare-ups, as well as to avoid triggers. Treatment falls into three parts:

1. Avoiding irritants
2. Moisturizing correctly
3. Using anti-inflammatory treatments such as steroid creams.

There are other more powerful treatments that may be offered by a skin specialist, including treatments that suppress the immune system, biological drugs and light therapy, but these are beyond the scope of this book, and fortunately the vast majority of patients with eczema will not need them.

Avoiding irritants: Try to follow the guidelines given below.

- Avoid soap, bubble baths and perfumed products, which can dry out the skin, but ask your doctor to prescribe your child a moisturizing soap-substitute. Plain water is also drying.
- When drying after a bath, gently pat your child's skin with a towel and do not rub.
- Use a non-biological washing powder.
- Use 100 per cent cotton clothing to allow your child's skin to 'breathe'.
- Prevent overheating: children with eczema get hot quickly, so dressing in thin layers can help. They should also sleep in an environment that is not too hot.
- Bathe your child using lukewarm water.

Moisturizing: In a child with eczema moisturizer should be applied at least once daily, even when their skin looks fine. The ideal time for moisturizing is right after bathing, to help lock the moisture in place – it's called 'soak and seal'. Bathing should not last more than five to ten minutes and the water temperature should be lukewarm. You may hear your doctor talk about applying an 'emollient': this is the medical word for a moisturizer, but these are different from the cosmetic moisturizers you may buy, as they are unperfumed and do not contain 'anti-ageing' ingredients.

<u>Top tip: 'Natural' doesn't always mean better</u>
Natural oils should be avoided as moisturizers in
children with eczema or those who are at risk of food
allergy. Despite its popularity, using olive oil as a
moisturizer is both damaging and increases allergen
absorption.[4] Instead, if your child has eczema, use
a non-oil-based eczema cream or ointment (your
family doctor can advise, if you are unsure) and
avoid moisturizers containing allergenic foods.

When you moisturize, apply a thick enough layer to see
it. By the time you are done, according to paediatric allergist
Dr Helen Brough, 'your child should look a bit like a snow-
man!' The moisturizer can take up to ten minutes to soak in.
Guidelines recommend that a large tub (about 500g/18 oz)
of a non-oil-based moisturizer (always use a moisturizer over
a lotion) should be used each week in children with eczema.

<u>Top tip: how to apply a moisturizing cream in eczema</u>
1. Wash your hands before applying the moisturizer,
   to prevent food and bacteria being transferred
   onto your child's skin.
2. Always avoid putting your hands inside pots of
   moisturizer, to reduce bacteria getting into the
   container. If the container becomes contaminated
   it will increase the risk of your child developing
   infected eczema. Instead, use a clean spoon to
   decant the moisturizer onto a clean plate, ready
   for use. Alternatively use a cream with a pump
   attached.

3. Hold the moisturizer in your hands for a few seconds to warm it, then moisturize reasonably fast, so that your child does not get cold. Apply to the skin in a downward direction following the hair growth, and allow time for it to soak in. Don't rub, as this could irritate the skin.

Steroid creams: These are available on prescription and will help reduce inflammation, but you need to follow your doctor's advice in using the correct amount and method of application. Although parents of children and other adults feel nervous about using steroid creams, they are safe to use, even in infants. Just squeeze some onto the length of your fingertip and apply a thin layer onto red and inflamed skin **only**, to avoid damaging the surrounding healthy skin. This is called a 'fingertip unit'. Most tubes have a standard 5mm nozzle, and one fingertip unit of cream should be sufficient to cover an area the size of your two hands.

Leave at least thirty minutes between applying a steroid and a moisturizer. Different doctors have different opinions on which should go on first, but to be honest, so long as you do both, that is the main thing. Strong steroid creams should be avoided on the face, neck and groin unless prescribed by a specialist.

Can you prevent eczema by moisturizing your baby's skin?

Not uncommonly by six months of age a baby can have multiple food allergies, and this is strongly associated with the presence of eczema. According to the dual-allergen exposure hypothesis (see page 24), if eczema could be prevented, this would lead to a significant reduction in food allergy. This led researchers to ask if there was a way to prevent eczema developing, and could something as simple as preventative moisturizing make a difference?

The Barrier Enhancement for Eczema Prevention (BEEP) study was published in March 2020.[5] More than 1,300 infants took part and, in a body blow, researchers found that moisturizing made no difference in **preventing** eczema (although it is still a crucial part of treating eczema once it has developed).In fact it increased parent-reported skin infections. There was also a small increase in food allergy (milk, egg, peanut) at two years of age in the active moisturizing group. This wasn't statistically significant, but it was disconcerting, to say the least. Since then the results of all the moisturizing and prevention eczema studies have been analysed in a process called a Cochrane Review. This is an independent analysis of data, to a very high level, and the disappointing conclusion is that daily moisturizing in healthy infants who do not have eczema does not prevent it and probably increases the risk of skin infection.[6]

Numerous other measures have also been tried to prevent eczema, including vitamin D supplements, giving children probiotics containing 'good bacteria' to tilt the gut microbiome away from allergy, and elimination diets in both mother and baby. None have worked, perhaps unsurprisingly, because we know that eczema is a complex, multifactorial, largely genetic disease.

So is food-allergy prevention all doom and gloom as well?

Preventing food allergy

When I began my allergy training, guidance from the Department of Health was to avoid peanut and other allergenic foods in children with a family history of allergy, until a child hit three years of age. There was no evidence for this, but the advice was based on what was thought to be the best option. Then, in 2015, everything changed, following publication of the Learning Early About Peanut Allergy (LEAP) study, which turned this conventional wisdom on its head.

What is the LEAP study?

Some years earlier Professor Gideon Lack, a professor of paediatric allergy at King's College London, had observed that peanut allergy was almost non-existent in Israeli children, compared to Jewish children in the UK who suffered from the allergy[7] about ten times as frequently.[8] The difference was that almost all infants in Israel were eating a peanut-containing snack called Bamba when they were teething during infancy – so from as early as four to six months of life. This was different from their British counterparts. He decided, along with senior co-investigator, Professor George Du Toit, to explore this further.

Some 640 children at medium or high risk of developing peanut allergy were recruited and split into two groups. Some were introduced to peanut in their diet before twelve months of age and were asked to keep eating it (three teaspoons of peanut butter per week); regular consumption is important. Others were advised to avoid peanut. The children were then followed until they were five years old and were fed peanut periodically, under hospital supervision, to determine if they had developed a peanut allergy. The results were quite startling. At the age of five there was an 81 per cent reduction in peanut allergy in those who were eating peanut consistently, compared to those who avoided it. Just over a year later the same group published again (the LEAP-ON study) and showed that when the original children in LEAP who did not develop peanut allergy took a break from eating peanut for a year, and then reintroduced it, they still did not react.[9] This second study was critical, as it demonstrated definitively that this was a prevention strategy.

Since the LEAP and LEAP-ON studies, the early introduction of egg has also been shown to help prevent allergy, but the formulation of the egg matters. So if the egg is heated or cooked, it seems to work better than if a powder is used.[10] So there is this window of opportunity in the early months of life to establish tolerance, and the science has now evolved to show that we should be introducing allergenic foods to infants before one year of age, and ideally between four and six months if they are at high risk. It appears that the longer introducing allergenic foods is delayed in higher-risk children, the greater the chance that they will develop a food allergy.

About 95 per cent of the population will never have to worry about this, but in children with persistent eczema, they are giving us a strong signal that they are different and are at far higher risk of developing a food allergy.

There is some debate, in children with a known egg allergy (who are therefore at higher risk of developing a peanut allergy), whether any testing is needed before introducing peanuts. The US guidelines recommend doing a peanut IgE skin test or blood test before feeding those higher-risk babies. In contrast, in Australia screening is not advised. In the UK the guidance is less definitive, but parents are encouraged not to delay introducing foods because of a lack of access to testing.

We know anaphylaxis in infants under twelve months of age is incredibly rare, and delaying food introduction in susceptible children is likely to carry a greater risk of them developing a lifelong, life-threatening food allergy. So most paediatric allergists that I know strongly encourage the early introduction of allergenic foods, such as milk, egg and nuts (this should always be in a soft form to prevent choking) – from four months onwards, or as soon as babies can hold their head upright independently and show an interest in food – as this will push their immune system away from developing a life-threatening food allergy.

What about pre-packaged early 'weaning' products to prevent food allergy?

All allergists agree that early introduction of allergenic foods is the most important part of preventing food allergy in high-risk infants. In recent years commercially produced early 'weaning' foods have come onto the market. These are marketed on the basis that they contain one or more common food allergens. So should you use them? Many experts say no, for several reasons:

- The amount of the allergenic food will vary between products, and some will contain very tiny amounts of the allergenic food. There is no evidence that these tiny amounts will prevent allergy at all.
- These products cost more than the individual allergenic foods and do not have the same nutritional benefit as eating the whole food itself.
- As these products are multi-allergen-containing, if a child reacts, it may be very difficult to promptly identify the cause of the reaction and weaning may be considerably delayed.

All of the above led the BSACI to release a statement in August 2021 declaring: 'As experts in infant nutrition, we believe that these products represent an over-medicalization of infant feeding . . . which risks unnecessary expense and complication for parents and provides no nutritional benefit compared to consuming the potentially allergenic foods in their natural form.'[11]

If you want to know more about how to introduce foods into your child's diet before six months of age there is a link to the early-feeding guidelines on the BSACI website in the Further Reading and Resources section (see page 221). There you will also find advice on how to introduce an allergenic food, if someone else in the home has that same food allergy.

The bottom line, when introducing allergenic foods in high-risk infants, is: put it in the diet and keep it in the diet.

Can treating eczema prevent food allergy?

There is growing evidence that the longer an infant has eczema, the greater their chance of developing a food allergy, particularly in the first twelve months of life. We also know that childhood food allergy increases the odds of asthma during adulthood by nearly threefold.[12] So can promptly and aggressively treating eczema nip food allergy in the bud? A Japanese study found that proactively getting on top of eczema using steroid creams led to an almost 50 per cent reduction in the number of children developing a food allergy. This is just one study, and the whole question is now being explored in a huge US/UK study called SEAL (Stopping Eczema and Allergy Study), which is expected to report back in 2027.

Breastfeeding versus bottle-feeding

Breastfeeding has many benefits for both mother and baby. We also know that the microbiome of children who are breast-fed is different from those who are bottle-fed, and that babies who go on to develop allergy have reduced microbial diversity, including fewer bifidobacteria and lactobacilli (another 'friendly' bacterium). However, we are still in the very early days in our understanding of the gut microbiome, and there is insufficient evidence for or against using breastfeeding to prevent food allergy in infants and young children.[13]

Diet in pregnancy

Lots of effort has been made to try and determine if there is any link between diet during pregnancy and a risk of allergy, but the data is inconsistent. An unhealthy diet is generally to be discouraged, whether someone is pregnant or not, but it would be a push to say we have proven that diet clearly links to the microbiome and to allergic disease. Furthermore, women do not need to avoid nuts and other allergenic foods, for fear of increasing their chances of having an allergic child. Trials looking at probiotics (live bacteria supplements) have, disappointingly, not shown a consistent improvement in reducing food allergy, although this may reflect the trial design itself, rather than probiotics having no merit.

The dos and don'ts of avoiding childhood allergy

Do:
- **Introduce solid foods** into your baby's diet from four months of age if they are at high risk of food allergy, if they have eczema (especially if it is severe) or already have a food allergy – provided they are ready. Include cooked egg and then peanuts (for example, smooth peanut butter; never the whole nut), followed by other foods known to cause food allergies. Once an allergenic food is introduced, it is important to keep it in your baby's diet on a consistent basis.

- **Eat whatever you want during pregnancy** – that includes allergenic foods such as milk, egg, peanuts or shellfish.

What not to do:
- **Do not eliminate foods from your baby's diet** without expert advice. If you feel you absolutely have to eliminate foods, you must reintroduce them two weeks later to see if your baby's eczema worsens once more. If there is no **clear** deterioration on reintroduction, then your baby does not have a delayed food allergy.
- **Do not eat nuts while breastfeeding** if your child has eczema, because 'nut dust' may drop onto your baby's skin, and experts think this may increase the odds of them developing a nut allergy.
- **Do not replace cow's milk** with goat's, sheep or buffalo milk; the proteins are too similar if your child is allergic.
- **Do not use soya protein formula** in the first six months of life to try and prevent food allergy.
- **Do not use olive oil or other natural oils** to moisturize your baby's skin.
- **Do not clean your baby's dummy using antiseptic**, as it leads to higher rates of proven food allergy.[14] We believe that the very small amounts of disinfectant that are swallowed skew the child's microbiome towards allergy.

Conclusion: Understanding Allergy

It feels fitting to end this expert guide with allergy prevention. While we may not have cracked the code when it comes to allergies, we are closer than ever to understanding how to prevent allergic disease and there are several exciting trials in the pipeline.

Every allergist – me included – longs for the day when we no longer see teenagers in our clinic with complex allergic disease that has plagued them since infancy. And although eliminating allergies may be impossible, reducing the numbers affected by them does not feel like an impossible dream. I believe that in the next decade our understanding will continue to grow, particularly as we unpick the microbiome and learn how to help it help us. The challenge then will be to convert this understanding into practical public-health measures.

Work is also proceeding at pace as researchers continue to explore allergy prevention. 'Hard' water has been shown to be linked to the development of eczema in many countries.[1] In infants carrying a mutation in the filaggrin gene, hard water increases their risk of developing eczema by almost three-fold.[2] So could water-softeners help prevent eczema? This is the very question that UK-based researchers are trying to answer, and the results are expected soon. Studies are also under way exploring diet in pregnancy and different weaning strategies and their impact on allergy risk. All of the above leaves me in little doubt that allergy prevention will continue to be an exciting space.

Then there are the relatively newer therapies like omalizumab and dupilumab, both man-made antibodies. Omalizumab (trade name Xolair) is licensed for patients who have moderate to severe persistent allergic asthma, despite conventional treatments. It is injected and targets IgE antibodies. It has been shown to reduce the severity and frequency of asthma exacerbations and to limit emergency hospital visits.[3] It is also licensed to treat chronic non-allergic urticaria, and its role in food immunotherapy and food allergy is being explored.[4] It has been approved for use in more than ninety countries to treat moderate to severe asthma, including the US, the EU, UK, Australia and New Zealand. However, access continues to be limited due to the significant cost.

In addition there is much excitement about dupilumab (tradename Dupixent). This drug, which is administered as an injection, reduces allergic inflammation by blocking two signalling proteins called interleukin-4 and interleukin-13. These interleukins worsen eczema by enhancing inflammation and exacerbating the already-leaky skin barrier. Dupilumab significantly reduces the severity of eczema in those in whom conventional treatments have not worked.[5] It is equally effective in white, Asian and Black/American racial groups[6] and is approved for use in more than sixty countries, including the US, Europe, the UK, Australia, New Zealand, Japan and China. It has also been approved for the treatment of severe asthma. Trials to evaluate its benefits in patients who suffer from both eczema and food allergy are underway.

Looking to the future, we are already starting to make huge leaps on the journey towards not only treating symptoms once they have occurred, but also using powerful drugs such as dupilumab to treat the root cause of allergy. At the same time we are learning more about how to prevent allergic disease. And new formulations of adrenaline may also not be far away, including an adrenaline nasal spray for the treatment of anaphylaxis.

I know that many people struggle for months or even years without access to specialist help. I am very aware that those who live with food allergy have to find ways to cope with an ever-present risk. I hope this book has equipped all those living with allergies with the knowledge, confidence and coping strategies to have more control over their own health. My goal is an ambitious one: I want people with allergies across the world to realize that often they do not need to suffer, and that there are new treatments. I hope this book will empower both you and your loved ones to lead a full, happy and healthy life.

A better understanding of allergy is what patients, their families, doctors and allergy specialists all want. This book is one very small part of that.

Appendix 1: Avoiding Individual Food Allergens

Whether you yourself have a food allergy or know someone who does, this appendix contains some basic information about common allergenic foods. Arranged in alphabetical order, these lists are not exhaustive but cover some common pitfalls. If you don't already, you must get into the habit of reading the label every time you purchase a food.

The bottom line is: if you are not confident about what a food contains, don't eat it.

Celery
- If you are allergic to celery, also avoid celeriac, which has similar allergens.
- The sticks, leaves and seeds (used to make celery salt) of celery can all be used and may be found in summer salads, soups and stews. Stock cubes and spice mixes may also contain celery. The yeast spread Marmite contains natural celery flavouring, although other yeast extracts may not; and tomato ketchup may also contain celery. It may also be added to batter and some cured bacon.
- Other considerations: cooking celery does not reduce its allergenicity, but small amounts may be tolerated as an ingredient in ketchup and other foods.

Cow's milk

- Main allergenic proteins: α-lactoglobulin, β-lactoglobulin, lactoferrin and casein.[1] If you are allergic to α-lactoglobulin or β-lactoglobulin you are likely to outgrow your milk allergy, but this is less likely to happen if you are sensitized to casein.

- Names in food: casein or caseinates, curd, ghee, hydrolysates, lactalbumin, lactalbumin phosphate, protein powders, recaldent, rennet, whey. However, these foods will usually be labelled with the word 'milk' either in bold or in brackets in the EU and the UK.

- Cross-reactivity with other animal milks: sheep, buffalo and goat's milk share similar proteins to cow's milk and are likely to trigger a reaction in those with CMPA.

- Other considerations: buttermilk or yoghurt is frequently used as a marinade for chicken or meat dishes. Dairy is often hidden in sausages, hot dogs and luncheon meats. Pesto sauce contains cheese. 'Vegan' does not automatically mean dairy-free, due to the risk of cross-contamination. Exercise caution in delicatessens, where cheese and meat may be sliced on the same machine. High-protein drinks will often contain milk proteins, so check the ingredients carefully. Dark chocolate is also problematic, due to the high risk of cross-contamination, as milk chocolate is often prepared on the same line. Before buying a dark-chocolate product, contact the manufacturer and check there is no risk of cross-contamination. Popcorn in cinemas may also he problematic as butter popcorn can easily cross contaminate plain.

Fish

- Main allergenic proteins: allergic reactions to finned fish are mainly caused by a protein called parvalbumin and, as it is found in many fish species, cross-reactivity between different fish groups is relatively common. Parvalbumin is not destroyed during the cooking process, so you can react to both raw and cooked fish. It can also be aero-solized.[2] This is why patients who are allergic to fish may react when they are in an environment where fish is being cooked, even if they do not eat it.
- Many fish-allergic children develop tolerance around ado-lescence, and most fish-allergic children can consume tuna and swordfish (as they contain very low levels of parval-bumin), which provide safe alternatives for a balanced diet.
- Other considerations: anchovies in particular can be tricky to avoid. Check for anchovy in: i) Caesar salad and Caesar dressing; ii) lamb dishes, where it may be used as a tender-izer; iii) pizza and pasta dishes; iv) Worcestershire sauce, and any barbeque sauces where Worcestershire sauce is an ingredient. Fish sauce is just that and is used widely in oriental cooking and to flavour kimchi. Seafood sticks (sometimes called crab sticks) are usually made from white fish. Fish can also be an ingredient in baby formula and in vitamins and foods that are enriched with added fish oil, although if you choose foods marked as vegetarian, these will be fish-free.

If you are allergic to fish are you likely to be allergic to shellfish?

Allergy to finned fish (such as cod and anchovies) and shellfish are often mentioned in the same breath, but they are two distinct allergies. However, care must be taken to avoid cross-contact – for example, when buying from the fish counter.

Hen's egg

- Main allergenic proteins: ovomucoid, ovalbumin, conalbumin and lysozyme. Individuals who are sensitized to egg white and ovamucoid are less likely than others to outgrow their egg allergy.[3]

- Names in food: Powdered/dried egg, egg proteins, including albumin (egg white), ovalbumin (a protein found in egg white), globulin, ovoglobulin, livetin, ovomucin, ovovitellin and vitellin.

- Cross-reactivity: likely with quail, duck and goose eggs and they should be avoided.

- Other considerations: eggs are widely used and will turn up in unexpected places. They are often used as a binding ingredient in everything from coating fish or chicken in breadcrumbs, to helping to shape meatballs. Beware of egg in prawn crackers, where it is used as a binding agent for tapioca, and in seafood/crab sticks (see page 193). Lysozyme can be found in some Italian hard cheeses, such as Grana Padano, and pasta may be made with egg. Most desserts contain egg. Check for it in royal icing, ice-cream, sweets and chocolate. 'Vegan' does not automatically mean egg-free, due to the risk of cross-contamination, so you must contact the company to check. Steer clear of shiny foods: sticky buns, pies and pasties may look irresistible in the window of your local bakery, but the chef has probably used an egg-based glaze to give it a glossy appearance.

Lupin beans

- Like peanut, the lupin is a member of the legume family and can be made into a flour. In some cases eating lupin can cause a reaction upon first exposure for someone with an existing legume allergy. Studies show that people with a peanut allergy have an increased chance of being also allergic to lupin, but this allergy nonetheless remains relatively uncommon. Therefore if you are allergic to peanuts, and if you are concerned, you can ask your family doctor to refer you for allergy testing. However, many of my patients read food labels scrupulously as a matter of course and prefer simply to avoid it.
- Foods to watch out for: lupin can be present in pasta, crepes and noodles, meat products like burgers and sausages, and baked goods such as bread and pastries. It is used to give them a yellow 'natural' look and is commonly added to gluten- and soya-free foods.

Mustard

- Mustard can be a difficult allergen to avoid. Its uses extend beyond the bottles of yellow sauce that we see on supermarket shelves. All parts of the mustard plant are likely to cause reactions in mustard-allergic individuals.

- Foods to watch out for: mustard seed and mustard oil are often used in Indian cooking, including curries. Mustard seeds and flowers, sprouted mustard seeds and mustard cress may be found in salads and sandwiches. In addition it can be found in mayonnaise, barbecue sauce, marinades and processed meats.

Peanut

- Although its name contains 'nut', peanut is a legume. It is also known as monkey nut. These are foods that grow in pods and include peanuts, peas, chickpeas, lentils, lupin, soya and beans.
- Main allergenic proteins: there are thirteen proteins in peanuts thought to cause a reaction, known as Ara h 1–13. It is estimated that more than 95 per cent of peanut-allergy patients are sensitized to at least one of the allergens Ara h 1, 2 and 3.[4] Ara h 2 is one of the dominant peanut allergens and sensitization is associated with ana-phylaxis; your allergist can check which specific peanut protein you are allergic to, if required.[5]
- Foods to watch out for: confectionery, cakes and vegetar-ian products are most likely to contain peanuts. Curries, Thai, Indonesian and other Eastern dishes are high-risk because many of them contain peanuts and their presence may not be obvious if the food is spicy. Beware of satay sauce, which is made from peanut.
- Other considerations: unrefined peanut oils, which may be called groundnut oil, may still contain allergenic peanut proteins and should be avoided if you have a peanut

allergy. It is often used in South-East Asian food. Refined peanut oil is generally considered safe for most people with a peanut allergy, because most (if not all) of the protein is removed during the manufacturing process. However, do discuss it with your doctor first. It's also worth noting that some fast-food chains such as Five Guys and the US chain Chick-fil-A use refined peanut oil for frying.

Sesame

- This is a flowering plant that produces edible seeds.
- Names in food: benne, benne seed, benniseed, gingelly, gingelly oil, sesamol, sesamolina, sesamum indicum, sim sim and tahini.
- Some allergic patients tolerate whole sesame seeds and only react to the crushed seeds, but if you are allergic, most allergists will advise complete avoidance.
- Foods with sesame: sesame seeds and oil are widely used in Asian and Middle Eastern dishes and may pop up unexpectedly – for example, in jerky. Sesame oil is made by cold-pressing sesame seeds, meaning that it retains its allergenicity and must be avoided. Be especially careful with salad dressing. Sesame-containing foods include crackers, breads, burger buns, salads, cereal bars, hummus (which contains a ground sesame paste called tahini) and falafel, plus rice and noodle soups.
- Other considerations: take 'may contain' sesame warnings on food seriously. It is a difficult allergen to control as it is small and 'clingy' and therefore may stick to surfaces.

Shellfish

- Main allergenic protein: tropomyosin – a protein also found in HDM, but there are many other allergenic proteins in shellfish allergy.
- Shellfish can be classified into crustaceans and molluscs. Crustaceans include crab, crayfish, langoustine, lobster and prawns. Molluscs include:

  1. Bivalves: mussels, oysters, scallops, clams
  2. Gastropods: limpets, periwinkles, snails
  3. Cephalopods: squid, cuttlefish, octopus.

- Cross-reactivity: if you are allergic to one shellfish, you are more likely to be allergic to another shellfish in the same group – prawns and crab (both crustaceans), for example – but may tolerate shellfish from a different group. However, to be certain you will need allergy investigation.
- Other considerations: be careful with fish dishes, as shellfish may be used to make a sauce, stock and scampi (which is made from a type of lobster). The basis of oyster sauce is boiling oysters in water for a long time; it is frequently used in Chinese cooking and is likely to be added to dishes such as noodle stir-fries, chow mein and beef with stir-fried vegetables. Fish sauce can also be made from shellfish. Be careful of squid ink, which may be used to colour risotto, pasta and other foods a deep black colour.

Can I take supplements if I have a fish or shellfish allergy?

Glucosamine supplements are common supplements taken to support joint health and are manufactured using the outer coating of a shellfish, so they should be avoided. Fish-oil supplements are also popular for heart and joint health. While the risk of allergic reactions to fish oils is thought to be low because of the purification process, check with your doctor before trying fish-oil supplements.

Soya

- Soya foods are made from the soya-bean plant, which is a member of the legume family.
- Names in foods: bean curd, edamame beans, hydrolyzed vegetable protein (HVP), miso, soy/soya, soya-protein isolate, soya protein / soya-protein products, soya albumin, soya bean, soya flour, soya milk, tempeh, textured vegetable protein (TVP), tofu.
- Foods with soya: soya can be ground down to make a flour that is added to breads, cakes, pasta and breakfast cereals.
- Soya milk is frequently found in body-building drinks.
- Other considerations: the increasing popularity of plant-based diets means that many people are looking for alternative protein sources than meat or fish, and so the market for soya-containing foods is burgeoning. Soya is found as mince, burgers and sausages, as well as being used in yoghurts and desserts as an alternative to dairy. It is also used as a filler in vegan, vegetarian and meat

products. Soya is a staple of Asian cooking, in the form of fermented soya foods such as tofu and unfermented soya foods, including miso and tempeh.

> ### Soya lecithin (E322)
> **The amount of soya protein that can contaminate the additive soya lecithin is so low that it is undetectable using current detection methods. Therefore most allergists do not even advise their soya-bean-allergic patients to avoid soybean lecithin when it is included as an ingredient on food products.**

Tree nuts

- These are nuts that grow on trees and include almonds, brazil nuts, cashew nuts, pistachio nuts, hazelnuts, macadamia nuts, pecan nuts and walnuts.
- Pine nuts and coconut are **not** tree nuts. Neither is nutmeg.
- Cross-reactivity: those with an existing peanut allergy have an up to 40 per cent chance of developing a tree-nut allergy, as similar proteins are found in both types. People who are allergic to cashew nuts are often (but not always) allergic to pistachio nuts, and those who are allergic to walnuts are invariably allergic to pecan nuts.
- Foods with tree nuts: confectionery, cakes, chocolates and ice-creams carry a high risk of containing nuts either as ingredients or as traces. In Indian, Far Eastern and Middle Eastern dishes nuts are widely used. I have seen pesto

sauce catch out many patients – cashew nuts are often used as a cheaper substitute for pine nuts.

- Other considerations: if you are already eating certain tree nuts without symptoms but are unsure about others, continue to eat the tree nuts that you are tolerating regularly, to prevent developing an allergy.

Wheat

- Main allergenic proteins: albumin, globulin, gliadins and glutenins.
- Foods to watch out for: wheat is the key ingredient of a range of foods, including breads, pasta, breakfast cereals, cakes, pancakes and pizzas. It is also used to make batter and is frequently found in convenience foods such as ready meals, soups, sauces and canned goods (a common example is the cornflour in baked beans) and as hydrolyzed wheat protein in processed meats. I have also seen patients get caught out by rusk – usually made from wheat – in sausages.
- Other considerations: gluten-free is not the same as wheat-free. Gluten-free foods are **not** safe for people with a wheat allergy.
- When foods are sold as gluten-free they are safe for people with coeliac disease, an autoimmune condition where the body reacts to gluten – a protein found in grains, including wheat, rye and spelt.
- Elevated levels of specific IgE to omega-5-gliadin are seen in wheat dependent exercise-induced anaphylaxis.

Appendix 2: Questions to Ask Your Doctor

When it comes to medical appointments, it pays to be prepared, and that can be hard when you are feeling anxious about your health or are desperate for answers. Here are some useful questions to help you stay calm and focused, whether you are visiting a doctor for the first time about a suspected allergy or attending a follow-up appointment.

At your family doctor's surgery

Before going to your appointment take a few minutes to think about what you want to get out of it. Prioritize your concerns: don't bring up something really important right at the end of the consultation. Briefly list the main problem and your troublesome symptoms (including the impact on your quality of life).

You should also ask your doctor:

- What is my treatment plan?
- Can I book a follow-up appointment now?
- What should I do if my symptoms don't get better, or they get worse?

If your doctor orders any blood tests, ask how you can get a copy of the results for your records. If you are referred to a specialist clinic, ask your family doctor what they are putting in their referral letter, so that you can ensure this covers all the points and is as detailed as possible – ask for a copy, and read the letter carefully.

Most allergy clinics will ask you to stop your antihistamines four days in advance of testing, to prepare for it. Other medicines, however, such as nasal steroid sprays or asthma pumps, should not be stopped.

Also ask your doctor how long the wait is to be seen by a specialist.

> ### Tips for preparing for a tele-medicine consultation
>
> Prepare for a tele-medicine consultation ahead of time, just as you would for a face-to-face appointment.
>
> 1. Are there questionnaires your allergist wants you to fill out beforehand?
> 2. Find somewhere quiet – do not have your consultation in a car while driving or in a busy public place.
> 3. Have your current list of prescribed medications to hand.
> 4. If you have small children, try to arrange childcare if possible, so that you can focus on talking to the doctor without being distracted.
> 5. Have details of any prior evaluation with allergy specialists that you may have had (you may be able to email these in advance) and any test results.

6. **If it is a younger child who is the patient, they do not need to be visible onscreen throughout the whole appointment.**

Visiting a specialist allergy clinic

If you were previously seen in a hospital, take a copy of your discharge summary, if you have one. Also bring a list of any allergy test results that your family doctor may have checked (if you have them) and either bring a prescription listing your regular medications or the medicines themselves.

What to take away

A first visit can feel overwhelming as you may leave with a lot of information, particularly if you have food allergy, rhinitis and asthma. So ask your specialist where to go to for more information: 'Have you got any leaflets, websites or local support groups you can direct me to?' You want reliable materials that you can take home and read at your leisure.

Make sure you are clear about follow-up appointments and who they are with. In my clinic we frequently refer patients on for further support with our nurse specialists and a dietician, as well as to see the doctor again.

Notes

Introduction

1 Foods Matter (2010), *Mintel's Allergy and Allergy Remedies UK*, www. foodsmatter.com/allergy_intolerance/miscellaneous/articles/mintel_allergy_report_2010.html
2 EAACI Advocacy Manifesto pdf, June 2015 version
3 R. S. Gupta, C. M. Warren, B. M. Smith, J. A. Blumenstock et al. (2018), 'The public health impact of parent-reported childhood food allergies in the United States', *Pediatrics*, 142 (6), e20181235, doi.org/10.1542/peds.2018-1235
4 P. J. Turner, D. E. Campbell, M. S. Matosue and R. L. Campbell (2020), 'Global Trends in Anaphylaxis Epidemiology and Clinical Implications', *Journal of Allergy and Clinical Immunology: In practice*, 8(4), pp. 1169–76

1. What Are Allergies and Why Do They Matter?

1 T. Zuberbier, J. Lötvall, S. Simoens et al. (2014), 'Economic burden of inadequate management of allergic diseases in the European Union: A GA(2) LEN review', *Allergy*, 69 (10), pp. 1275–9
2 R. Gupta, A. Sheikh, D. P. Strachan and H. R. Anderson (2004), 'Burden of allergic disease in the UK: Secondary analyses of national databases', *Clinical & Experimental Allergy: Journal of the British Society for Allergy and Clinical Immunology*, 34 (4), pp. 520–26, doi.org/10.1111/j.1365-2222.2004.1935.x
3 R. S. Gupta et al. (2019), 'Prevalence and Severity of Food Allergies Among US Adults', *Journal of the American Medical Association Network Open*, 2 (1), e185630, 4 January 2019, doi.org/10.1001/jamanetworkopen.2018.5630
4 A. M. Wattseta (2021), 'The Gut Microbiome of Adults with Allergic Rhinitis is Characterised by Reduced Diversity and an Altered Abundance of Key Microbial Taxa Compared to Controls', *International Archives of Allergy and Immunology*, 182 (2), pp. 94–105

2. The Allergy Epidemic

1 J. Bostock (1819), 'Case of a Periodical Affection of the Eyes and Chest', *Medico-Chirurgical Transactions*, 10 (1), pp.161–5

2 B. I. Nwaru, L. Hickstein, S. S. Panesar et al. (2014), 'Prevalence of common food allergies in Europe: A systematic review and meta-analysis', *Allergy*, 69 (8), pp.992–1007

3 EAACI Advocacy Manifesto pdf, June 2015 version

4 American College of Allergy, Asthma and Immunology (2018), 'Allergy Facts', acaai.org/news/facts-statistics/allergies

5 N. J. Osborne et al. (2011), 'Prevalence of challenge-proven IgE-mediated food allergy using population-based sampling and pre-determined challenge criteria in infants', *Journal of Allergy and Clinical Immunology*, 127, pp.668–76

6 S. Singh, B. B. Sharma, S. Salvi et al. (2018), 'Allergic rhinitis, rhinoconjunctivitis, and eczema: Prevalence and associated factors in children', *Clinical Respiratory Journal*, 12 (2), pp.547–56

7 X.-Y. Wang et al. (2018), 'Prevalence of pollen-induced allergic rhinitis with high pollen exposure in grasslands of northern China', *Allergy*, 73 (6), pp.1232–43

8 A. B. Conrado et al. (2021), 'Food anaphylaxis in the United Kingdom: Analysis of national data, 1998–2018', *British Medical Journal* (Clinical research edn), 372 (251), doi.org/10.1136/bmj.n251

9 H. A. Suaini et al. (2021), 'Children of Asian ethnicity in Australia have higher risk of food allergy and early-onset eczema than those in Singapore', *Allergy*, doi.org/10.1111/all.14823

10 R. J. Buka et al. (2015), 'Anaphylaxis and ethnicity: Higher incidence in British South Asians', *Allergy*, 70 (12), pp.1580–87

11 A. E. Clarke et al. (2021), 'Demographic characteristics associated with food allergy in a Nationwide Canadian Study', *Allergy, Asthma, and Clinical Immunology: Official Journal of The Canadian Society of Allergy and Clinical Immunology*, 17 (1), doi.org/10.1186/s13223-021-00572-z

12 M. E. Levin et al. (2020), 'Environmental factors associated with allergy in urban and rural children from the South African Food Allergy (SAFFA) cohort', *Journal of Allergy and Clinical Immunology*, 145 (1), pp.415–26

13 T. Marrs et al. (2019), 'Dog ownership at three months of age is associated with protection against food allergy', *Allergy*, 74 (11), pp.2212–19

14 P. J. Turner et al. (2020), 'Global Trends in Anaphylaxis Epidemiology and Clinical Implications', *Journal of Allergy and Clinical Immunology: In Practice*, 8 (4), pp.1169–76

15 K. Yamamoto-Hanada et al. (2017), 'Influence of antibiotic use in early childhood on asthma and allergic diseases at age 5', *Annals of Allergy, Asthma &Immunology: Official publication of the American College of Allergy, Asthma, & Immunology*, 119 (1), pp.54–8

16 A. G. Hirsch, J. Pollak, T. A. Glass et al. (2017), 'Early-life antibiotic use and subsequent diagnosis of food allergy and allergic diseases', *Clinical & Experimental Allergy*, 47 (2), pp.236–44

17 S. Metzler, R. Frei, E. Schmaußer-Hechfellner et al. (2019), 'Association between antibiotic treatment during pregnancy and infancy and the development of allergic diseases', *Pediatric Allergy and Immunology*, 30 (4), pp.423–33

18 B. Darabi et al. (2019), 'The association between caesarean section and childhood asthma: An updated systematic review and meta-analysis', *Allergy, Asthma & Clinical Immunology: Official Journal of the Canadian Society of Allergy and Clinical Immunology*, 15 (62), doi.org/10.1186/s13223–019–0367–9

19 J. Gerlich et al. (2018), 'Pregnancy and perinatal conditions and atopic disease prevalence in childhood and adulthood', *Allergy*, 73 (5), pp.1064–74, doi.org/10.1111/all.13372

20 V. X. Soriano et al. (2021), 'Infant pacifier sanitization and risk of challenge-proven food allergy: A cohort study', *Journal of Allergy and Clinical Immunology*, 147 (5), pp.1823–9

21 H. A. Brough et al. (2013), 'Peanut protein in household dust is related to household peanut consumption and is biologically active', *Journal of Allergy and Clinical Immunology*, 132 (3), pp.630–38

22 G. Lack et al. (2003), 'Factors associated with the development of peanut allergy in childhood', *The New England Journal of Medicine*, 348 (11), pp.977–85

3. Runny Nose and Itchy Eyes: Understanding Hay Fever and Rhinitis

1 V. Bauchau and S. R. Durham (2004), 'Prevalence and rate of diagnosis of allergic rhinitis in Europe', *European Respiratory Journal*, 24 (5), pp.758–64

2 P. J. Bousquet, B. Leynaert, F. Neukirch et al. (2008), 'Geographical distribution of atopic rhinitis in the European Community Respiratory Health Survey I, *Allergy*, 63 (10), pp.1301–9

3 J. Bousquet, N. Khaltaev, A. A. Cruz et al. (2008), 'Allergic Rhinitis and its Impact on Asthma (ARIA) 2008 update (in collaboration with the World Health Organization, GA(2)LEN and AllerGen)', *Allergy*, 63 (86), pp.8–160

4 C. R. Roxbury, M. Qiu, J. Shargorodsky et al. (2019), 'Association Between Rhinitis and Depression in United States Adults', *Journal of Allergy and Clinical Immunology: In Practice*, 7 (6), pp.2013–20

5 M. K. Church and T. Zuberbier (2019), 'Untreated allergic rhinitis is a major risk factor contributing to motorcar accidents', *Allergy*, 74 (7), pp. 1395–7

6 D. H. Mudarri (2016), 'Valuing the Economic Costs of Allergic Rhinitis, Acute Bronchitis, and Asthma from Exposure to Indoor Dampness and Mold in the US', *Journal of Environmental and Public Health*, 2386596, doi.org/10.1155/2016/2386596

7 A. Shah, R. Pawankar (2009), 'Allergic rhinitis and co-morbid asthma: Perspective from India ARIA Asia-Pacific Workshop report', *Asian Pacific Journal of Allergy and Immunology*, 27 (1), pp.71–7

8 W. R. L. Anderegg, J. T. Abatzoglou, L. D. L. Anderegg et al. (2021), 'Anthropogenic climate change is worsening North American pollen seasons', *Proceedings of the National Academy of Sciences of the USA*, 118 (7), e2013284118, doi.org/10.1073/pnas.2013284118, doi.org/10.1073/pnas.2013284118

9 A. Kurganskiy, S. Creer, N. de Vere et al. (2021), 'Predicting the severity of the grass pollen season and the effect of climate change in Northwest Europe', *Science Advances*, 7 (13), eabd7658, doi.org/10.1126/sciadv.abd7658

10 G. D'Amato, L. Cecchi, S. Bonini et al. (2007), 'Allergenic pollen and pollen allergy in Europe', *Allergy*, 62 (9), pp.976–90

11 U. Schaffner, S. Steinbach, Y. Sun et al. (2020), 'Biological weed control to relieve millions from Ambrosia allergies in Europe', Nature Communications, doi.org/10.1038/s41467-020-15586-1

12 To find out more about this, see: www.rcpch.ac.uk/resources/inside-story-health-effects-indoor-air-quality-children-young-people#what-changes-are-needed

13 S. Walker et al. (2007), 'Seasonal allergic rhinitis is associated with a detrimental impact on exam performance in UK teenagers: case-control study', *Journal of Allergy and Clinical Immunology*, 120 (2), pp.381–7

14 F. Thien, P. Beggs, D. Csutoros et al. (2018), 'The Melbourne epidemic thunderstorm asthma event 2016: An investigation of environmental triggers, effect on health services, and patient risk factors', *Lancet Planetary Health*, 2 (6), pp.255–63

15 Asthma Australia (2020), 'Asthma First Aid', asthma.org.au/what-we-do/how-we-can-help/first-aid/

16 M. A. Schei, J. O. Hessen and E. Lund (2022), 'House-dust mites and mattresses', *Allergy: European Journal of Allergy and Clinical Immunology*, 57 (6), pp.538–42

17 J. D. Miller (2019), 'The Role of Dust Mites in Allergy', *Clinical Reviews in Allergy And Immunology*, 57 (3), pp.312–29

18 E. R. Tovey, M. D. Chapman and T. A. Platts-Mills (1981), 'Mite faeces are a major source of house dust allergens', *Nature*, 289 (5798), pp. 592–3

19 D. W. Vredegoor, W. Doris et al. (2012), '*Can f 1* levels in hair and homes of different dog breeds: Lack of evidence to describe any dog breed as hypoallergenic', *Journal of Allergy and Clinical Immunology*, 130 (4), pp. 904–9

20 E. Satyaraj, C. Gardner, I. Filipi et al. (2019), 'Reduction of active Fel d1 from cats using an anti Fel d1 egg IgY antibody', *Immunity Inflammation and Disease*, 7, pp. 68–73

4. Please Make It Stop: Treating Rhinitis and Hay Fever

1 D. Rabago and A. Zgierska (2009), 'Saline nasal irrigation for upper respiratory conditions', *American Family Physician*, 80 (10), pp. 1117–19

2 The Met Office, 'What is the pollen count?', www.metoffice.gov.uk/weather/warnings-and-advice/seasonal-advice/health-wellbeing/pollen/what-is-the-pollen-count

3 A. B. Ozturk, E. Celebioglu, G. Karakaya and A. F. Kalyoncu (2013), 'Protective efficacy of sunglasses on the conjunctival symptoms of seasonal rhinitis', *International Forum of Allergy & Rhinology*, 3 (12), pp. 1001–6

4 I. Terreehorst et al. (2003), 'Evaluation of impermeable covers for bedding in patients with allergic rhinitis', *The New England Journal of Medicine*, 349 (3), pp.237–46

5 S. Y. Choi et al. (2008), 'Optimal conditions for the removal of HDM, dog dander, and pollen allergens using mechanical laundry', *Annals of Allergy, Asthma & Immunology*, 100 (6), pp.583–8

6 J. M. Wilson and T. Platts-Mills (2018), 'Home environmental interventions for house dust mite', *Journal of Allergy and Clinical Immunology: In Practice*, 6 (1), pp.1–7

7 M. K. Church and D. S. Church (2013), 'Pharmacology of antihistamines', *Indian Journal of Dermatology*, 58 (3), pp.219–24

8 J. M. Weiler et al. (2000), 'Effects of Fexofenadine, Diphenhydramine, and Alcohol on Driving Performance: A Randomized, Placebo-Controlled Trial in the Iowa Driving Simulator', *Annals of Internal Medicine*, 132 (5), pp.354–63

9 S. L. Gray, M. L. Anderson, S. Dublin et al. (2015), 'Cumulative use of strong anticholinergics and incident dementia: A prospective cohort study', *Journal of the American Medical Association Internal Medicine*, 175 (3), pp.401–7

10 J. O. Warner (2001), 'ETAC Study Group. Early Treatment of the Atopic Child: A double-blinded, randomized, placebo-controlled trial of cetirizine in preventing the onset of asthma in children with atopic dermatitis: 18 months' treatment and 18 months' posttreatment follow-up', *Journal of Allergy and Clinical Immunology*, 108 (6), pp.929–37

11 G. K. Scadding et al. (2017), 'BSACI guideline for the diagnosis and management of allergic and non-allergic rhinitis (Revised Edition 2017; First Edition 2007)', *Clinical & Experimental Allergy*, 47 (7), pp.856–89

12 G. Passalacqua et al. (2007), 'Allergic rhinitis and its impact on asthma update: Allergen immunotherapy', *Journal of Allergy and Clinical Immunology*, 119 (4), pp.881–91, doi.org/10.1016/j.jaci.2007.01.045

13 S. R. Durham et al. (1999), 'Long-term clinical efficacy of grass-pollen immunotherapy', *The New England Journal of Medicine*, 341 (7), pp.468–75

5. COVID-19 and Allergy

1 Scientific Advisory Group for Emergencies (2021), 'VEEP: Vaccine effectiveness table, 16 July 2021', www.gov.uk/government/publications/veep-vaccine-effectiveness-table-16-july-2021

2 D. Logunov et al. (2020), 'Safety and immunogenicity of an rAd26 and rAd5 vector-based heterologous prime-boost COVID-19 vaccine in two formulations: Two open, non-randomised phase 1/2 studies from Russia', *The Lancet*, doi.org/10.1016/S0140-6736(20)31866-3

3 S. Lovinsky-Desir et al. (2020), 'Asthma among hospitalized patients with COVID-19 and related outcomes', *Journal of Allergy and Clinical Immunology*, 146 (5), pp.1027–34

4 R. Strauss, N. Jawhari, A. M. Attaway et al. (2021), 'Intranasal Corticosteroids Are Associated with Better Outcomes in Coronavirus Disease 2019', *Journal of Allergy and Clinical Immunology: In Practice*, 9 (11), pp. 3934–40.e9

5 L. B. Robinson et al. (2021), 'COVID-19 severity in hospitalized patients with asthma: A matched cohort study', *Journal of Allergy and Clinical Immunology: In Practice*, 9 (1), pp.497–500

6 A. A. Dror, N. Eisenbach, T. Marshak et al. (2020), 'Reduction of allergic rhinitis symptoms with face mask usage during the COVID-19 pandemic', *Journal of Allergy and Clinical Immunology: In Practice*, 8 (10), pp.3590–93

7   M. Greenhawt, E. M. Abrams, M. Shaker et al. (2021), 'The Risk of Allergic Reaction to SARS-CoV-2 Vaccines and Recommended Evaluation and Management: A Systematic Review, Meta-Analysis, GRADE Assessment, and International Consensus Approach', *Journal of Allergy and Clinical Immunology: In Practice*, S2213–2198(21)00671–1, doi.org/10.1016/j.jaip.2021.06.006

8   M. S. Krantz et al. (2021), 'Anaphylaxis to the first dose of mRNA SARS-CoV-2 vaccines: Don't give up on the second dose!', *Allergy*, doi. org/10.1111/all.14958

6. An Introduction to Food Allergies

1   A. Muraro et al. (2014), 'EAACI food allergy and anaphylaxis guidelines: Diagnosis and management of food allergy', *Allergy*, 69 (8), pp.1008–25

2   C. Venter et al. (2008), 'Prevalence and cumulative incidence of food hypersensitivity in the first 3 years of life', *Allergy*, 63 (3), pp.354–9

3   J. Li, L. M. Ogorodova, P. A. Mahesh et al. (2020), 'Comparative study of food allergies in children from China, India, and Russia: The EuroPrevall-INCO surveys', *Journal of Allergy and Clinical Immunology: In Practice*, 8 (4), pp.1349–58

4   European Academy of Allergy and Clinical Immunology (EAACI) (2014), 'Food Allergy & Anaphylaxis Public Declaration', dgaki.de/ wp-content/uploads/2014/04/FoodAllergyAnaphylaxisPublicDeclarationCombined.pdf

5   S. Voltolini et al. (2014), 'New risks from ancient food dyes: Cochineal red allergy', *European Annals of Allergy and Clinical Immunology*, 46 (6), pp. 232–3

6   Rachel L. Peters et al. (2018), 'The Prevalence of Food Sensitization Appears Not to Have Changed between 2 Melbourne Cohorts of High-Risk Infants Recruited 15 Years Apart', *Journal of Allergy and Clinical Immunology: In Practice*, 6 (2), pp.440–48

7   A. Baseggio Conrado et al. (2021), 'Food anaphylaxis in the United Kingdom: Analysis of national data, 1998–2018', *British Medical Journal* (Clinical research edn), 372, n.251, doi.org/10.1136/bmj.n251

8   Ibid.

9   S. Dua et al. (2019), 'Effect of sleep deprivation and exercise on reaction threshold in adults with peanut allergy: A randomized controlled study', *Journal of Allergy and Clinical Immunology*, 144 (6), pp. 1584–94

10 A. Nowak-Węgrzyn (2015), 'What makes children outgrow food allergy?', *Clinical & Experimental Allergy*, 45 (11), pp.1618–20

7. Stranger than Fiction: Food Allergies You May Not Have Heard Of

1 I. J. Skypala, S. Bull, K. Deegan et al. (2013), 'The prevalence of PFS and prevalence and characteristics of reported food allergy: A survey of UK adults aged 18–75 incorporating a validated PFS diagnostic questionnaire', *Clinical & Experimental Allergy*, 43 (8), pp.928–40

2 S. Wagner and H. Breiteneder (2002), 'The latex-fruit syndrome', *Biochemical Society Transactions*, 30 (6), pp.935–40

3 R. M. Maulitz et al. (1979), 'Exercise-induced anaphylactic reaction to shellfish', *Journal of Allergy and Clinical Immunology*, 63 (6), pp.433–4

4 B. Minty (2017), 'Food-dependent exercise-induced anaphylaxis', *Canadian Family Physician / Le Médecin de famille canadien*, 63 (1), pp.42–3

5 R. A. Bansal et al. (2021), 'The first reported cases of meat allergy following tick bites in the UK', *Journal of the Royal Society of Medicine Open*, 12 (4); doi.org/10.1177/2054270421996131

6 To find out more about this, see: www.cdc.gov/lyme/prev/on_people.html

7 S. Scheurer et al. (2021), 'The Role of Lipid Transfer Proteins as Food and Pollen Allergens Outside the Mediterranean Area', *Current Allergy and Asthma Reports*, 21 (2), doi.org/10.1007/s11882-020-00982-w

8. Delayed Food Allergies

1 D. Munblit et al. (2020), 'Assessment of Evidence About Common Infant Symptoms and Cow's Milk Allergy', *Journal of the American Medical Association Pediatrics*, 174 (6), pp.599–608

2 S. Khan, X. Guo, T. Liu et al. (2021), 'An Update on Eosinophilic Esophagitis: Etiological Factors, Coexisting Diseases, and Complications', *Digestion*, 102 (3), pp.342–56

3 Ibid.

4 P. Navarro et al. (2019), 'Systematic review with meta-analysis: The growing incidence and prevalence of eosinophilic oesophagitis in children and adults in population-based studies', *Alimentary Pharmacology & Therapeutics*, 49 (9), pp.1116–25

5 J. K. Harris, R. Fang, B. D. Wagner et al. (2015), 'Esophageal microbiome in eosinophilic esophagitis', *PloS One*, 10 (5), e0128346

6 G. T. Furuta and D. A. Katzka (2015), 'Eosinophilic Esophagitis', *The New England Journal of Medicine*, 373 (17), pp.1640–48

7 Ibid.

8 M. V. Lenti et al. (2021), 'Diagnostic delay and misdiagnosis in eosinophilic oesophagitis', *Digestive and Liver Disease: Official Journal of the Italian*

Society of Gastroenterology and the Italian Association for the Study of the Liver, doi.org/10.1016/j.dld.2021.05.017

9 D. Melgaard et al. (2021), 'A diagnostic delay of 10 years in the DanEoE cohort calls for focus on education – a population-based cross-sectional study of incidence, diagnostic process and complications of eosinophilic oesophagitis in the North Denmark Region', *United European Gastroenterology Journal*, 9 (6), pp.688–98

10 J. D. Hamilton, S. Harel, B. N. Swanson et al. (2021), 'Dupilumab suppresses type 2 inflammatory biomarkers across multiple atopic, allergic diseases', *Clinical & Experimental Allergy*, 51 (7), pp.915–31

11 Y. Katz and M. R. Goldberg (2014), 'Natural history of food protein-induced enterocolitis syndrome', *Current Opinion in Allergy and Clinical Immunology*, 14 (3), pp.229–39

9. How Will I Cope? – Living with a Food Allergy

1 Food Standards Agency (2021), 'Food Allergy and Intolerance', www.food.gov.uk/safety-hygiene/food-allergy-and-intolerance

2 Ibid.

3 National Allergy Research Foundation, 'Natasha's Law', www.narf.org.uk/natashaslaw

4 Anaphylaxis Campaign, 'Airline Allergy Policies', www.anaphylaxis.org.uk/living-with-anaphylaxis/travelling/airline-allergy-policies

5 Department for Education (2020), 'Allergy Guidance for Schools', www.gov.uk/government/publications/school-food-standards-resources-for-schools/allergy-guidance-for-schools

6 Allergy UK, 'Whole-School Allergy Awareness and Management', www.allergyuk.org/information-and-advice/for-schools/whole-school-allergy-awareness-management

10. Anaphylaxis: Reducing the Fear – What You Should Know

1 P. Turner et al. (2020), 'Global Trends in Anaphylaxis Epidemiology and Clinical Implications', *Journal of Allergy and Clinical Immunology: In Practice*, 8 (4), pp.1169–76

2 R. S. H. Pumphrey and M. H. Gowland (2007), 'Further fatal allergic reactions to food in the United Kingdom, 1999–2006', *Journal of Allergy and Clinical Immunology*, 119 (4), pp.1018–19

3 E. M. Abrams, A. G. Singer, L. Lix et al. (2017), 'Adherence with epinephrine autoinjector prescriptions in primary care', *Allergy, Asthma & Clinical Immunology*, 13 (46), doi.org/10.1186/s13223–017–0218–5

4 L. Noimark et al. (2012), 'The use of adrenaline autoinjectors by children and teenagers', *Clinical and Experimental Allergy: Journal of the British Society for Allergy and Clinical Immunology*, 42 (2), pp.284–92

5 D. M. Fleischer et al. (2012), 'Allergic reactions to foods in preschool-aged children in a prospective observational food allergy study', *Pediatrics*, 130 (1), e25–32, doi.org/10.1542/peds.2011–1762

6 Anaphylaxis Campaign, 'Take the Kit', www.anaphylaxis.org.uk/campaigning/takethekit/

7 www.epipen.co.uk; www.jext.co.uk; auvi-q.com; www.emerade.com

8 C. L. M. Joseph, A. R. Sitarik, R. Kado et al. (2021), 'Sesame allergy is more prevalent among Middle Eastern/North African patients in an urban healthcare system', *Journal of Allergy and Clinical Immunology: In Practice*, S2213–2198(21)00663–2, doi.org/10.1016/j.jaip.2021.05.036

9 H. C. Y. Lam et al. (2021), 'Seasonality of food-related anaphylaxis admissions and associations with temperature and pollen levels', *Journal of Allergy and Clinical Immunology: In Practice*, 9 (1), pp.518–20.e2

10 R. G. Lambley (2021), 'Human donor milk also protects against severe retinopathy of prematurity', *British Medical Journal* (Clinical research edn), 372 (25), doi.org/10.1136/bmj.n25

11 C. Brooks, A. Coffman, E. Erwin and I. Mikhail (2017), 'Diagnosis and treatment of food allergic reactions in pediatric emergency settings', *Annals of Allergy, Asthma & Immunology*, 119 (5), pp.467–8

11. Taking the Medicine: The Importance of Drug Allergies

1 P. J. Turner et al. (2017), 'Fatal Anaphylaxis: Mortality Rate and Risk Factors', *Journal of Allergy and Clinical Immunology: In Practice*, 5 (5), pp.1169–78

2 R. Mirakian et al. (2015), 'Management of allergy to penicillins and other beta-lactams', *Clinical & Experimental Allergy*, 45 (2), pp.300–27

3 R. M. West et al. (2019), '"Warning: allergic to penicillin": Association between penicillin allergy status in 2.3 million NHS general practice electronic health records, antibiotic prescribing and health outcomes', *Journal of Antimicrobial Chemotherapy*, 74 (7), pp.2075–82

4 National Institute for Health and Care Excellence (2014), 'Drug allergy: Diagnosis and management', www.nice.org.uk/guidance/cg183

5 R. Warrington et al. (2018), 'Drug allergy', *Allergy, Asthma & Clinical Immunology*, 14 (2), doi.org/10.1186/s13223–018–0289-y

6 E. Macy and R. Contreras (2014), 'Health care use and serious infection prevalence associated with penicillin "allergy" in hospitalized patients:

A cohort study', *Journal of Allergy and Clinical Immunology*, 133 (3), pp. 790–96

7 West et al. (2019), '"Warning: allergic to penicillin", *Journal of Antimicrobial Chemotherapy*, 74 (7), pp.2075–82

8 L. W. Kaminsky, S. Dalessio, T. Al-Shaikhly and R. Al-Sadi (2021), 'Penicillin allergy label increases risk of worse clinical outcomes in COVID-19', *Journal of Allergy and Clinical Immunology: In Practice*, doi.org/10.1016/j.jaip.2021.06.054

9 M. Couto et al. (2012), 'Selective anaphylaxis to paracetamol in a child', *European Annals of Allergy and Clinical Immunology*, 44 (4), pp.163–6

10 Royal College of Anaesthetists, 'Anaesthesia, Surgery and Life-Threatening Allergic Reactions', www.nationalauditprojects.org.uk/NAP6Report?newsid=1914#pt

12. Red Herrings: When You Think You Are Allergic . . . But You Aren't

1 N. P. Conlon, A. Abramovitch, G. Murray et al. (2015), 'Allergy in Irish adults: A survey of referrals and outcomes at a major centre', *Irish Journal of Medical Science*, 184 (2), pp.349–52

2 J. Fricke et al. (2020), 'Prevalence of chronic urticaria in children and adults across the globe: Systematic review with meta-analysis', *Allergy*, 75 (2) pp.423–32

3 R. J. Powell, S. C. Leech, S. Till et al., 'British Society for Allergy and Clinical Immunology: BSACI guideline for the management of chronic urticaria and angioedema', *Clinical & Experimental Allergy*, 45 (3), pp. 547–65

4 W. Vleeming et al. (1998), 'ACE inhibitor-induced angioedema: Incidence, prevention and management', *Drug Safety*, 18 (3), pp.171–88

5 T. Brown et al. (2017), 'Angiotensin-converting enzyme inhibitor-induced angioedema: A review of the literature', *Journal of Clinical Hypertension*, 19 (12), pp.1377–82

14. Turning Off the Tap: Eczema and Allergy Prevention

1 M. Yumiko et al. (2020), 'Earlier aggressive treatment to shorten the duration of eczema in infants resulted in fewer food allergies at 2 years of age', *Journal of Allergy and Clinical Immunology: In Practice*, 8 (5), pp. 1721–4

2 O. Tsilochristou, G. du Toit, P. H. Sayre et al. (2019), 'Association of *Staphylococcus aureus* colonization with food allergy occurs independently of eczema severity', *Journal of Allergy and Clinical Immunology*,

144 (2), pp.494–503, doi10.1016/j.jaci.2019.04.025, doi.org/:10.1016/j.jaci.2019.04.025

3 Skin Deep, www.dftbskindeep.com

4 D. Y. M. Leung et al. (2021), 'Olive oil is for eating and not skin moisturization', *Journal of Allergy and Clinical Immunology*, S0091–6749(21)00813–7, doi.org/10.1016/j.jaci.2021.04.037

5 J. R. Chalmers et al. (2020), 'Daily emollient during infancy for prevention of eczema: The BEEP randomised controlled trial', *The Lancet*, 39510228, pp.962–72, doi.org/10.1016/S0140–6736(19)32984–8

6 M. M. Kelleher et al. (2021), 'Skin care interventions in infants for preventing eczema and food allergy', *Cochrane Database of Systematic Reviews*, 2 (2), CD013534, doi.org/10.1002/14651858.CD013534.pub2

7 G. Du Toit, Y. Katz, P. Sasieni et al. (2008), 'Early consumption of peanuts in infancy is associated with a low prevalence of peanut allergy', *Journal of Allergy and Clinical Immunology*, 122 (5), pp.984–91

8 I. A. Myles, C. R. Castillo, K. D. Barbian et al. (2020), 'Therapeutic responses to Roseomonas mucosa in atopic dermatitis may involve lipid-mediated TNF-related epithelial repair', *Science Translational Medicine*, 12 (560), doi.org/10.1126/scitranslmed.aaz8631

9 G. Du Toit, P. H. Sayre, G. Roberts et al. (2016), 'Effect of Avoidance on Peanut Allergy after Early Peanut Consumption', *The New England Journal of Medicine*, 374 (15), pp.1435–43

10 M. R. Perkin, K. Logan, A. Tseng et al. (2016), 'Randomized Trial of Introduction of Allergenic Foods in Breast-Fed Infants', *The New England Journal of Medicine*, 374 (18), pp.1733–43

11 British Society for Allergy and Clinical Immunology (2021), 'Position Statement on Pre-packaged early weaning products marketed to prevent food allergies', www.bsaci.org/wp-content/uploads/2021/08/Position-Statement-on-Pre-docx.pdf?mc_cid=395030d10f&mc_eid=0b41762b8a

12 W. C. G. Fong, A. Chan, H. Zhang et al. (2021), 'Childhood food allergy and food allergen sensitisation are associated with adult airways disease: A birth cohort study', *Pediatric Allergy and Immunology*, doi.org/10.1111/pai.13592

13 S. Halken et al. (2020), 'EAACI guideline: Preventing the development of food allergy in infants and young children (2020 update)', *Pediatric Allergy and Immunology*, 32 (5), pp.843–58

14 V. X. Soriano, J. J. Koplin, M. Forrester et al. (2021), 'Infant pacifier sanitization and risk of challenge-proven food allergy: A cohort study', *Journal of Allergy and Clinical Immunology*, 147 (5), pp.1823–9

Conclusion: Understanding Allergy

1 Z. K. Jabbar-Lopez, C. Y. Ung, H. Alexander et al. (2021), 'The effect of water hardness on atopic eczema, skin barrier function: A systematic review, meta-analysis', *Clinical & Experimental Allergy*, 51(3), pp.43–51

2 Z. K. Jabbar-Lopez, J. Craver, K.Logan et al. (2020), 'Longitudinal analysis of the effort of water hardness on atopic eczema', *British Journal of Dermatology*, 183(2), pp.285–93

3 M. Humbert et al. (2005), 'Benefits of omalizumab as add-on therapy in patients with severe persistent asthma who are inadequately controlled despite best available therapy (GINA 2002 step 4 treatment): INNOVATE', *Allergy*, 60 (3), pp.309–16

4 N. A. Hanania et al. (2011), 'Omalizumab in severe allergic asthma inadequately controlled with standard therapy: A randomized trial', *Annals of Internal Medicine*, 154 (9), pp.573–82

5 E. L. Simpson et al. (2016), 'Two Phase 3 Trials of Dupilumab versus Placebo in Atopic Dermatitis', *The New England Journal of Medicine*, 375 (24), pp.2335–48

6 A. F. Alexis et al. (2019), 'Efficacy of Dupilumab in Different Racial Subgroups of Adults With Moderate-to-Severe Atopic Dermatitis in Three Randomized, Placebo-Controlled Phase 3 Trials', *Journal of Drugs in Dermatology*, 18 (8), pp.804–13

Appendix 1: Avoiding Individual Food Allergens

1 L. Jaiswal and W. Mulumebet (2021), 'Recent perspective on cow's milk allergy and dairy nutrition', *Critical Reviews in Food Science and Nutrition*, doi.org/10.1080/10408398.2021.1915241

2 A. Dahlman-Höglund, A. Renström, F. Acevedo and E. Andersson (2013), 'Exposure to parvalbumin allergen and aerosols among herring processing workers', *Annals of Occupational Hygiene*, 57 (8), pp.1020–29

3 K. M. Jarvinen, K. Beyer, L. Vila et al. (2007), 'Specificity of IgE antibodies to sequential epitopes of hen's egg ovomucoid as a marker for persistence of egg allergy', *Allergy*, 62 (7) pp.758–65

4 H. Chassaigne, I. V. Nørgaard, A. J. Hengel (2007), 'Proteomics-based approach to detect and identify major allergens in processed peanuts by capillary LC-Q-TOF (MS/MS)', *Journal of Agricultural and Food Chemistry*, 55 (11), pp.4461–73

5 O. Hemmings, G. Du Toit, S. Radulovic et al. (2020), 'Ara h 2 is the dominant peanut allergen despite similarities with Ara h 6', *Journal of Allergy and Clinical Immunology*, 146 (3), pp.621–30

Glossary

Below is a list of abbreviations and frequently used terms.

AAI: Adrenaline autoinjector

AIT: Allergen immunotherapy, a treatment that changes the way the immune system reacts to allergens by switching off the allergy; it is therefore also known as desensitization

Allergen: A harmless substance such as pollen or peanut, triggering an allergic reaction

Allergy: This occurs when the immune system reacts to a substance that is usually harmless to most people

Anaphylaxis: A rapid-onset, severe allergic reaction leading to either breathing difficulties or low blood pressure; the first-line treatment is always adrenaline

Asthma: A common condition where the lower airways become inflamed and narrowed, obstructing the flow of air into and out of the lungs; common symptoms include wheezing, shortness of breath, difficulty breathing, chest tightness and cough (especially at night); common triggers include allergies, cold viruses, exercise and cigarette smoke

Atopy: A genetic tendency to develop allergic disease, so that your immune system is more likely to produce IgE antibodies to common allergens. Examples of atopic conditions include asthma, rhinitis and eczema

BSACI: British Society for Allergy & Clinical Immunology

CMPA: Cow's milk protein allergy

Drug challenge: A procedure where increasing amounts of a particular drug are given to a person while under allergist supervision; it is very commonly used in drug allergy

EAACI: European Academy of Allergy and Clinical Immunology

Eczema: A group of inflammatory conditions of the skin, which can make the skin red, itchy and more prone to infection and dryness; in brown or black skin, grey or violet-brown discoloration is often seen rather than red rashes

EoE: Eosinophilic oesophagitis – inflammation of the oesophagus, leading to difficulty swallowing and food getting stuck; it is an immune condition that is caused by a build-up of white blood cells called eosinophils

Food challenge: A procedure where increasing amounts of a particular food are fed to a person while under medical supervision; it is normally used by allergy specialists to determine whether or not a patient is allergic to a food

Food intolerance: A broad term to describe a reaction to a food that is not caused by the immune system; rarely dangerous, and more common than a food allergy, intolerance symptoms usually occur because the body is not properly digesting food

FPIES: Food protein-induced enterocolitis is a severe condition where inflammation in the gut is triggered by a delayed food allergy

HDM: House dust mite

ICS: Inhaled corticosteroid, used as a preventative treatment in asthma

IgE: Immunoglobulin E, the class of antibodies that causes immediate allergic reactions

IgE-mediated allergy: Allergic reactions caused by the IgE antibody

IgG: Immunoglobulin G, the most common type of antibody found in the circulation of blood and extra-cellular fluid; it primarily protects the body from viral, bacterial and fungal infection and does not cause allergic responses or food intolerance. Successful allergen immunotherapy is associated with an increase in allergen-specific IgG.

LTP allergy: Lipid transfer protein allergy is so named after the type of proteins in fruits, vegetables, nuts, seeds and cereals that an allergic person is sensitized to

Microbiome: All of the genetic material within the microbiota

Microbiota: The community of bacteria, viruses and fungi that live within a particular environment – in the context of this book, within us

NHS: The UK's National Health Service

Non-IgE-mediated allergy: Allergic reactions that are not caused by the IgE antibody; skin-prick tests are not helpful in their diagnosis

NSAID: Non-steroidal anti-inflammatory drug, part of a group of painkillers that include aspirin, diclofenac and ibuprofen

Pathogen: microorganisms such as bacteria, viruses, fungi and parasites that can cause disease

Rhinitis: Inflammation of the lining of the nose

Sensitization: The presence of IgE antibodies to an allergen; some (but not all) individuals who are sensitized will go on to develop an allergy

Specific IgE test: A blood test to measure different IgE antibodies targeted against allergens, for example to pollens or foods; these tests help with (but in isolation do not make) an allergy diagnosis

WBC: white blood cell, also known as a leukocyte

Further Reading and Resources

General allergy charities (by country)

Australia: www.allergyfacts.org.au

Canada: www.allergyfoundation.ca

Europe: this page on the EAACI website will give you links to country-specific patient organizations in more than twenty nations: patients.eaaci.org/eaaci-member-patient-organisations/

New Zealand: www.allergy.org.nz

South Africa: Allergy Foundation South Africa, a non-profit organization offering patient advice and allergy training, www.allergyfoundation.co.za/

UK: Allergy UK charity, www.allergyuk.org
www.anaphylaxis.org.uk
beatanaphylaxis.co.uk

USA: Asthma and Allergy Foundation of America (AAFA), www.aafa.org

Allergic rhinitis and asthma (charities and professional organizations)

Europe: European Federation of Allergy and Airways Disease: a non-profit organization co-ordinating twenty-six European patient associations: www.efanet.org

European Forum for Research and Education in Allergy and Airway diseases, a non-profit organization with a patient information site, www.euforea.eu/patient-platform

Italy: Federation of Asthma and Allergy, a patient association, www.federasmaeallergie.org

Norway: Norwegian Asthma and Allergy Foundation, a healthcare and campaigning foundation with a national pollen alert, www.naaf.no

UK: Asthma UK, asthma.org.uk

USA: Allergy and Asthma Network, allergyasthmanetwork.org/

Eczema and food allergy (charities and professional organizations)

Canada: Food Allergy Canada, a non-profit organization, www.foodallergycanada.ca

Italy: www.foodallergyitalia.org
Netherlands: Food Allergy Foundation, www.voedselallergie.nl/
Portugal: www.alimenta.pt
UK: Anaphylaxis Campaign, UK charity, www.anaphylaxis.org.uk
Food Standards Agency, for advice on UK food-labelling laws, www.food.
    gov.uk/safety-hygiene/food-allergy-and-intolerance
Natasha Allergy Research Foundation, a UK charity set up by the family of
    Natasha Ednan-Laperouse, www.narf.org.uk
National Eczema Society, UK charity, www.eczema.org
USA: www.eczema.com
Food Allergy Research and Education, a US charity, www.foodallergy.org
US Food and Drug Administration, www.fda.gov

Food-allergy translation cards

Allergy Action, food-allergy translation cards, www.allergyaction.org
Equal Eats, food-allergy translation cards, www.allergytranslation.com

Adrenaline autoinjector (AAI) manufacturers

Auvi-Q, auvi-q.com
Emerade, www.emerade.com
Epipen, www.epipen.co.uk
Jext, www.jext.co.uk

Weaning

British Society for Allergy and Clinical Immunology, early-feeding
    guidelines, www.bsaci.org/professional-resources/resources/early-feeding-
    guidelines/

Podcasts

Conversations from the World of Allergy, the AAAAI, www.aaaai.org/
    Professional-Education/Podcasts
The Doctor's Kitchen, Dr Rupy Aujla covers general physical and mental-health
    topics, including allergy, www.thedoctorskitchen.com/podcasts
The Itch, with Dr Payel Gupta and Kortney Kwong Hing, who lives with mul-
    tiple food allergies, asthma and eczema, www.itchpodcast.com
Jason K. Lee, allergist and immunologist, www.soundcloud.com/jason-k-
    lee-364925682

Allergy professional organizations (by country)

Australia and New Zealand: Australasian Society of Clinical Immunology and Allergy, a professional body of allergists and clinical immunologists, www.allergy.org.au

Brazil: Brazilian Association of Asthma and Allergy, a professional organization, www.asbai.org.br

Europe: European Academy of Allergy & Clinical Immunology (EAACI), a non-profit association of clinicians, researchers and allied health professionals dedicated to improving the health of people affected by allergic diseases, www.eaaci.org

India: Indian College of Allergy, Asthma & Applied Immunology: icaai.net/

Pakistan: Asthma and Immunology Society, a professional organization, www.allergypaais.org

Saudi Arabia: Saudi Arabian Allergy and Asthma Society, a professional organization, www.saais.org.sa/en

UK: British Society for Allergy & Clinical Immunology, a national, professional and academic society, www.bsaci.org

USA: American Academy of Allergy, Asthma & Immunology, a professional medical association, www.aaaai.org

COVID-19 and vaccines

Australia and New Zealand: Australasian Society of Clinical Immunology and Allergy COVID-19 vaccination FAQs, www.allergy.org.au/patients/ascia-COVID-19-vaccination-faq

UK: Anaphylaxis Campaign COVID-19 advice, www.anaphylaxis.org.uk/COVID-19-advice/pfizer-COVID-19-vaccine-and-allergies/

UK government's Green Book information on vaccines and vaccination procedures, including for the COVID-19 vaccines, www.gov.uk/government/collections/immunisation-against-infectious-disease-the-green-book

US: American College of Allergy, Asthma & Immunology COVID-19 vaccine FAQs, www.acaai.org/news/frequently-asked-patient-questions-about-the-COVID-19-vaccine/

Johns Hopkins University open-access global tracker on COVID-19 statistics, coronavirus.jhu.edu/map.html

Acknowledgements

I 'always' knew I wanted to be a doctor, and when I was a child my father indulged this. We used to spend hours together in bookshops and he would patiently wait while I pored through books in the medical section. He died in January 2019, and I wish he could have known that one day his daughter would write a book that might be found in the very same bookshops that he had taken me to. He lived my medical dream with me and words of thanks are insufficient. I also want to thank my mother. She has always believed in me, been there for me and, despite battling advanced Parkinson's, has supported me in every way possible while I was writing this book. I am indebted to both my mother and father.

I want to publicly thank my mother's carers, Anna, Armanda, Maggie, Sara and Shellica, who have done everything to take care of her, so that I could focus on writing; and my family (especially Ismail and Munni Puppi) for being there for me throughout this process. I also want to mention my Italian 'family' for keeping me in olive oil and love while I have been writing. *Grazie mille*, Chiara. It's been a journey and you have all been my companions.

I want to acknowledge my medical and dietetic colleagues, both in the UK and abroad: Dr Zainab Abdurrahman, Dr Mayjay Ali, Dr Joanna Ball, Dr Bachi Begishvili, Dr Dave Christie, Dr Linda Dykes, Dr Claudia Gore, Dr Nicola Jay, Dr Helgi Johannsson, Professor Liz Lightstone, Dr Anna

Marquiss, Mrs Julia Marriott, Professor Florin-Dan Popesc, Dr Kate Prior, Dr Brian Schroer, Dr Isabel Skypala, Dr Paul Turner, Dr Carina Venter and Dr John Weiner have all inspired me or supported me in some way while writing the book. I especially want to thank my St Mary's colleagues, Dr Cecilia Trigg and Mrs Tanya Wright, whose shared passion for food allergy is infectious; as well as paediatric allergist Dr Helen Brough at the Evelina London Children's Hospital (Guy's and St Thomas's), for advising me on allergy prevention, delayed CMPA and the treatment of eczema; and Professor Dave Stukus at the Nationwide Children's Hospital in Ohio, for sharing with me his gems of paediatric-allergy common sense. Finally I must mention Professor Jonathan Bennett at the Glenfield Hospital, Leicester, who, despite fighting on the front line against COVID-19, has nonetheless found time to act as my sounding board. He has been unstinting in his time, advice and generosity of spirit. Every person mentioned here is a great clinician and I am lucky to know you all.

Of course a book does not get written without a team. Jaime Marshall, my agent, has been brilliant throughout. Jaime, I struck lucky meeting you, and thank-you will never be a big enough word. I also want to thank my editors, Lydia Yadi and Susannah Bennett, and the team at Penguin Random House, for giving me the chance to write this book and for introducing me to Kat Keogh, who as contributing editor is a marvel and has been a delight to work with.

Throughout the book there are case histories. I want to thank all my patients who have allowed me to share their stories – especially Kate and her daughter Emily, for allowing me to share their very personal experience of anaphylaxis.

My final thanks go to my patients and my followers on Twitter (especially Dan Barker, Wendy Russell Barter, Simon Lane, Justin Stach and Geoff White). Through your questions, your interaction and your messages you have shaped me into the allergist I am today.

You are, and will remain, my inspiration.

PREPARING FOR THE PERIMENOPAUSE AND MENOPAUSE

DR LOUISE NEWSON

The *Sunday Times* Number One Bestseller.

Part of the Penguin Life Experts series.

Dr Louise Newson is the UK's leading menopause specialist, and she's determined to help women thrive during the menopause.

Despite being something that almost every woman will experience at some point in their lives, menopause is frequently misdiagnosed and misinformation and stigma are commonplace. Dr Newson demystifies the menopause and explains why every woman should be perimenopause-aware, regardless of their age.

Using new research, expert advice and empowering patient stories from a diverse range of women who have struggled to secure adequate treatment and correct diagnosis, Dr Newson equips readers with expert advice and practical tips. She empowers women to confidently take charge of their health and their changing bodies.

It's never too early to learn about the perimenopause or menopause and this compact guide will provide you with everything you need to know.

MANAGING YOUR MIGRAINE
DR KATY MUNRO

Part of the Penguin Life Experts series.

Despite being one of the most common and debilitating conditions in the world, migraine is still widely misunderstood, stigmatized and misdiagnosed. Migraine is much more than 'just a headache', so why do we still know so little about this genetic neurological brain disorder and its causes? Headache specialist and GP Dr Katy Munro has the answers you're looking for.

Managing Your Migraine is the practical go-to guide for understanding migraine, equipping readers with practical, expert advice.

If you're a person with migraine, or know someone struggling, this book will provide helpful strategies for alleviating and managing your symptoms. Drawing on her medical expertise, her own personal experience with migraine and the stories of her patients, Dr Munro will empower you to get to know your own migraine and build an effective treatment plan that will help you to live your life to the full.

MANAGING IBS
DR LISA DAS

Part of the Penguin Life Experts series.

Irritable bowel syndrome is a complex and frustrating condition that is not yet fully understood but affects an astounding 10 per cent of the global population.

Unfortunately, IBS patients don't often get the right advice or support they need. Dr Lisa Das, UK-leading gastroenterologist and IBS specialist, offers practical, empowering and evidence-based advice on how to manage and treat the condition successfully.

KEEPING YOUR HEART HEALTHY
DR BOON LIM

Part of the Penguin Life Experts series.

One of the world's leading cardiologists, Dr Boon Lim, has created the go-to guide to keeping your heart in good shape for optimum health.

This concise, accessible book covers everything you need to know about improving and maintaining your heart health. From hypertension, cholesterol and inherited cardiac conditions, to chest pain, fainting and stress, Dr Lim draws on his years of knowledge and expertise to offer readers practical, easy-to-follow advice.

If you're experiencing heart problems, have high blood pressure or cholesterol, or think you or a loved one might be at increased risk of heart attack or stroke, this book will provide step-by-step tips on how to prevent and reduce heart issues by exercising more, being mindful of your nutrition and diet and by making smarter, healthier lifestyle choices.

This is the ultimate guide to your heart: how it works, when it struggles, what it needs to function optimally and how you can shape your lifestyle to keep it ticking for a long time.